D0770277

Table of Contents

Preface

Economics has changed the face of health care today. Economics is driving a system that is expensive and available to only a portion of the population. Hospital stays are costly, shorter and more technologically advanced. Individuals are being discharged both sicker and quicker. Because of these and other factors, homecare is playing an increasingly important role in health care. More specifically, in the area of cancer care, homecare has a unique role.

Cancer therapies are being given with increasing frequency on an outpatient basis and in the home setting. Homecare has a role in the care of people with cancer. This often-forgotten arena of health care, has a cadre of nurses with strong clinical skills, creativity, and a genuine interest in patient care.

Since cancer affects one in three individuals, it is likely that the nurse working in the home will care for a person with cancer. This manual was developed for nurses who provide care to persons with cancer in the home. It provides both the technological, as well as the practical therapies of home care. The manual covers current cancer-related topics in depth.

I have been a nurse for twenty years; most of those years I have worked with people with cancer. It has been my pleasure to gather a group of experts together and have them share their knowledge and expertise with you. I hope this book is a useful tool for all nurses, in particular, for those working in homecare.

Margaret Barton Burke, RN, MS, OCN

Overview of Cancer Care

Marcia C. Liebman, RN, MS, OCN
Oncology Clinical Nurse Specialist
Southwood Community Hospital, Norfolk, Massachusetts

OVERVIEW OF CANCER CARE

Marcia C. Liebman, RN, MS, OCN
Oncology Clinical Nurse Specialist
Southwood Community Hospital, Norfolk, Massachusetts

INTRODUCTION

Current cancer treatment many times consists of more than one kind of therapy. More and more cancers once treated by surgery alone are today being treated with various combinations of surgery, radiation therapy, chemotherapy, and biotherapy. Treatments from different modalities may be given consecutively or concurrently. Side effects may be intensified by multimodal therapy.

This section will cover principles of the various cancer treatment modalities, management of symptoms from both the disease and its treatment, and oncologic emergencies.

PRINCIPLES OF CANCER THERAPY

The goals of cancer therapy are cure, control, or palliation. Cure means that disease is eradicated and the patient will live his full life span and die of something other than cancer. Control means that the cancer is kept from spreading, i.e., a remission is induced and survival time is increased. Palliation is treatment for symptom control, i.e., radiation therapy for pain due to extensive bone metastasis.

The major cancer treatment modalities are surgery, radiation therapy, chemotherapy, and biotherapy. Surgery and radiation are local treatments, that is, they only affect a limited area—either the area that has been removed surgically or the area that has been radiated. Chemotherapy and biotherapy are systemic treatments; the goal is to affect cancer cells throughout the body.

Surgery

Surgery plays a major role in both the diagnosis and the treatment of cancer. The principle behind surgical treatment is to remove the diseased area from the body. Many times it is the treatment of choice for early cancer; unfortunately 50 70% of newly diagnosed patients already have micrometastasis, which means that surgery alone will not cure the patient. When surgery alone is not curative, it can play a major role in debulking the tumor, thus possibly increasing the effectiveness of the other treatment modalities.

Care for the person who has had surgical treatment of cancer is based on nursing practice learned in basic nursing programs. Post-operative healing has begun by the time a patient is discharged home. Home care for the cancer patient entails monitoring for complications, maintaining healing through adequate nutrition, preventing infection, and meeting psychosocial needs, including the need for information.

Radiation Therapy

Radiation therapy is usually used in conjunction with surgery or chemo-therapy and it may be used for curative, as well as palliative, reasons.

Because radiation is a local therapy, side effects occur only at the area being treated. Radiating the breast, for example, will not cause hair loss or nausea and vomiting. Radiation controls tumor growth by affecting cellular reproduction. Radiation can either be external or internal. The majority of external beam radiation patients are treated daily on an outpatient basis for four to six weeks. Internal radiation, also called brachytherapy, can be administered as an oral solution or as an implant. Patients receiving brachytherapy are usually hospitalized for a few days.

When a person is receiving external beam radiation, the treatment area is carefully determined so as to give the maximum effect with the minimum amount of radiation to healthy areas of the body. The radiation field is usually outlined in purple marker; sometimes permanent tiny tatoos are placed in the corners of the field. These marks should not be washed off and the area inside the marks need special attention, as it is at high risk for skin breakdown. Table 1.1 illustrates patient teaching points the homecare nurse should include in care of the person receiving radiation.

TABLE I.I

**Information for the Person Receiving
External Beam Radiation Therapy**

- avoid tight-fitting clothing in the treatment field. This especially includes bras, girdles, and belts.

- wear cotton clothing over the treatment field as much as possible. Cotton is soft and non-irritating and allows the skin to "breathe".

- use baby detergent on clothing worn over the treatment area to keep them soft and to avoid exposure to residue harsh detergents.

- protect the skin from sun exposure. This is both during and after completion of treatment.

- avoid heat to the skin, specifically hot water bottles, heating pads, and hot shower water.

- avoid swimming in salt water or chlorinated pools.

- avoid use of soap (use mild soap, if necessary), deodorants, lotions, or powders in the treatment area. If lotion is needed for dry skin, consult the radiation nurse or physician about specific products to use.

- use an electric razor if the area needs to be shaved.

- check the skin daily for signs of breakdown or infection.

Chemotherapy

Chemotherapy is the administration of chemicals which are known to kill cancer cells. Chemotherapy may be given orally, subcutaneously, intramuscularly, intravenously, intra-arterially, intrathecally, or into a body cavity. Chemotherapy is considered a systemic therapy with a wide range of side effects. Chemotherapeutic agents are usually not given as single agents, but are given in combinations so as to maximize the amount of cancer cell death, while sparing as many normal cells as possible. Chemotherapeutic regimens can be quite complex. Most chemotherapy is given on an outpatient basis; usually only persons with multiple health problems, severe debilitation, or continuous infusion chemotherapy are hospitalized. The development of ambulatory pumps and venous access devices has made home therapy possible for this last category of patients.

Different chemotherapeutic agents are given for different cancers; some agents work better on certain cancers than others. This sometimes confuses patients, as they expect to have the same reaction as their neighbor, who had a different kind of cancer and received different chemotherapy. Patients also respond differently to chemotherapy and two people on the same dose of the same drug may have different experiences.

Appendix 1 includes chemotherapeutic agents administered most frequently in the home setting. Care plans are identified for each agent.

Biotherapy

Biotherapy is the use of biological response modifiers (BRMs). BRMs can boost the immunologic mechanisms; have direct tumor activity; or have other biological effects, such as, interfering with the tumor cells' ability to metastasize. Biotherapy is a systemic treatment whose full range of uses has yet to be determined. This form of cancer treatment has begun to move into homecare. Appendix 2 is a glossary of terms used in biotherapy.

Two BRMs which are used in home therapy are interferon and colony stimulating factors. Interferons appear to have antiviral, antiproliferative, antitumor, and immunomodulatory effects. They may be useful in both hematological and solid malignancies; they may be used alone or in conjunction with chemotherapy.

An exciting kind of BRM, colony stimulating factors (CSFs), is not used as a cancer therapy but is used in combating the side effects of cancer therapy. CSFs stimulate the growth of blood cells in the bone marrow. Currently available are granulocyte-macrophage colony stimulating factor (GM-CSF), granulocyte colony stimulating factor (G-CSF), and erythropoietin (EPO). The first two stimulate growth of white blood cells and the last stimulates growth of red blood cells. The role of CSFs in cancer treatment is to counteract the bone marrow depression seen as a side effect of many chemotherapeutic agents. Many times the dose of chemotherapy is limited by its bone marrow toxicity; CSFs allow higher doses of chemotherapy to be given (if organ toxicity does not occur) and can also prevent the delay frequently seen when a scheduled antitumor treatment is held because the bone marrow has not yet recovered from the last treatment. CSF is usually given subcutaneously either daily or three times a week. It is started approximately 24 hours after the patient has received chemotherapy. CSF does not prevent bone marrow depression, but it decreases the time the bone marrow is depressed.

Currently, only GM-CSF and G-CSF are approved for use in cancer patients. EPO is approved for use in dialysis patients, patients with end-stage renal failure, and HIV positive patients on zidovudine. The drug has been supplied by the manufacturer for compassionate use in cases where religious convictions have prevented a patient from allowing blood transfusions.

Side effects commonly associated with biotherapy are flu-like symptoms, including headache, upper respiratory infection symptoms, fatigue, malaise, nausea, vomiting, and diarrhea; hypotension; somnolence and confusion; skin rash; bone marrow depression; and anaphylaxis.

Some general considerations when using BRMs include:

1. BRMs usually need to be refrigerated.

2. Different brands may have different doses. If the brand is changed, the dose may also have to be altered.

3. Anti-inflammatory drugs (such as ibuprofen) and steroids may interfere with the action of BRMs. Patients need to consult the oncologist before taking any medication. As ibuprofen is now an over-the-counter medication and can also be found in other over-the-counter medications, patients need to check all non-prescription drugs with their doctor or pharmacist.

SYMPTOM MANAGEMENT

Nursing care for the person with cancer requires management of side effects of therapy as well as of the disease itself. Symptom management has become nursing's role in cancer care. Nurses have developed expertise in this area, both in the hospital and at home.

Bone Marrow Depression

Bone marrow depression (BMD), also known as myelosuppression or bone marrow suppression, is the inhibition of bone marrow activity and is an expected side effect of most chemotherapeutic agents and of radiation therapy to areas where there is a large amount of bone marrow activity (i.e., the pelvis and the sternum). It is also an expected complication of some cancers.

Specific cells affected in BMD are leukocytes or white blood cells (WBCs), which fight infection; erythrocytes or red blood cells (RBCs), which carry oxygen; and thrombocytes or platelets, which are important for clotting. Chemotherapy and radiation therapy don't affect mature circulating cells, only those still developing in the bone marrow. This explains why it usually takes 10 to 14 days until the peripheral or circulating WBCs, RBCs, and/or platelets reach their "nadir" or lowest point: that is the time it takes developing cells to become mature circulating cells. It is important to understand that not all treatments cause BMD nor do they equally affect the cells in the bone marrow; cyclophosphamide, for instance, is "platelet sparing".

Complete blood counts (CBCs) are usually done weekly for people on chemotherapy and every one to two weeks for people receiving radiation therapy. By monitoring the CBC, the physician can determine if the next scheduled dose of therapy needs to be delayed and nurses can advise their patients as to when they are "at risk" for infection, fatigue, and/or bleeding.

Normal values of the CBC are shown in Table 1.2.

TABLE I.2

Complete blood count

Cell element	Normal value
white blood cells	5,000 - 10,000 cells/mm^3
neutrophils	50 - 70%
lymphocytes	20 - 40%
monocytes	2 - 6%
eosinophils	1 - 4%
basophils	0.5 - 1%
hemoglobin	14 - 16.5 g/dL (men)
	12 - 16 g/dL (women)
hematocrit	42 - 51% (men)
	37 - 47% (women)
platelets	140,000 - 400,000 cells/mm^3

Infection

When a person is leukopenic (has a WBC of less than 3,000 to 4,000), "infection precautions" are usually initiated and treatment may be delayed. There is controversy over whether someone with a WBC of less than 1,000 should be hospitalized and placed on "reverse" or "protective" precautions. It is generally believed that unless an infection already exists, the patient is less likely to become infected if he remains at home. The practice of putting on a gown and mask when entering the room of someone on protective precautions has also fallen into disuse, as studies have demonstrated that good handwashing is just as effective. Sometimes even a strictly protective environment is not adequate protection from infection; a severely neutropenic patient can become infected from the bacteria in his bowel. Nursing interventions for the person at risk for infection can be found in Table 1.3.

TABLE I.3

Nursing Interventions for the Leukopenic Patient

Teach "infection precautions" to patient/family as a preventative measure to be used when the WBC is less than 4,000. These are:

- avoid people with colds and avoid crowded places.
- take your temperature every evening (more often if you think it is needed). Report temperatures greater than 100° F to your physician.
- report signs and symptoms of infection: cough with or without sputum, fever, difficulty voiding, cloudy urine.
- achieve and maintain optimal nutritional status.
- maintain daily fluid intake of 3,000 ml unless contraindicated.
- conserve energy; get adequate rest.
- maintain good body hygiene; shower or bathe daily.
- wash hands frequently; avoid cracking of hands and other areas by applying lotion to dry, chapped areas.
- avoid rectal temperatures and enemas.
- avoid straining to expel stool. May need to use stool softeners.
- use a soft toothbrush and clean mouth after every meal and before bed.
- avoid cleaning bird cages, cat litter boxes, and areas containing dog excreta.
- avoid all sources of stagnant water. Have someone add 1 tsp chlorine bleach to each quart of water used in flower vases and 1 tsp vinegar to each quart of water or saline used in respiratory equipment.

Avoid the use of intermittent or indwelling catheters, if possible.

Care of the patient who has developed an infection is discussed in Section 4 (page 77) of this book.

Bleeding

"Bleeding precautions" are initiated when a person is thrombocytopenic (the platelet count is less than 50,000 to 100,000). The risk of spontaneous bleeding does not usually occur until the platelets are less than 20,000 and platelet transfusions may not be given to an asymptomatic person unless the platelet count is less than 20,000. Table 1.4 identifies nursing interventions for the patient with thrombocytopenia.

TABLE 1.4

Nursing Interventions for the Thrombocytopenic Patient

Teach bleeding precautions to patient/family as a preventative measure to be used when platelets are less than 100,000. These are:

- avoid trauma and tight fitting clothing.
- check skin daily for unexplained bruises.
- use an electric razor when shaving.
- keep skin moist and prevent cracking by using lubricants.
- avoid medications that contain aspirin.
- eat a high protein diet.
- use an emery board instead of nail scissors.

Test urine, stool, and vomitus for occult blood.

Coordinate/avoid invasive procedures, i.e., venipunctures, enemas,intramuscular injections.

For nosebleeds, place patient in high Fowler's position and apply ice to nape of neck and bridge of nose.

Administer platelets as ordered.

Fatigue

Fatigue can be caused by anemia, protein-calorie malnutrition, disruption of rest and sleep patterns, pain, stress, depression, or accumulation of waste products due to cellular destruction caused by therapy. Table 1.5 illustrates the nurse's role when caring for a person with fatigue.

TABLE I.5

Nursing Interventions for the Person with Fatigue

- Assess pattern of fatigue and determine cause of fatigue.
- Teach patient to schedule rest periods as needed, prioritize activities, and ask for assistance from others.
- Encourage patient to drink 3,000 ml of fluids daily to avoid accumulation of cellular waste products.
- Relieve pain.
- Assist patient to achieve and maintain optimal level of nutrition. Encourage a diet rich in iron, protein, Vitamin B12, and folic acid.
- Provide emotional support.
- Administer blood products as ordered.
- Administer oxygen as ordered.

Flu-like syndrome

This is a common syndrome seen with BRMs. Signs and symptoms are implicit in its name. Nursing intervention should include the assessment of the patient's symptoms in order to exclude infection, especially in patients who are neutropenic.

Premedicate with acetaminophen and antihistamine per physician's order. Avoid aspirin and anti-inflammatory agents unless specifically approved by the physician, as they interfere with the action of the BRMs. Encourage daily intake of 3,000 ml of fluids and allow for rest. Provide emotional support for the patient and family. Patient/family education about BRMs will help them know what to expect from therapy.

Gastrointestinal symptoms

Cancer and its therapy affect the gastrointestinal tract in multiple ways. Radiation to the head and neck can cause mucositis, stomatitis, and esophagitis, as well as taste changes. Radiation to the abdomen can cause nausea and vomiting. Radiation to the pelvis causes diarrhea. Chemotherapy can cause all these symptoms. It can also cause constipation, as can narcotics.

Nursing interventions for each of these symptoms are outlined in Table 1.6. *Eating Hints* (free from the National Cancer Institute) and is recommended for use by both the nurse and the patient to help most gastrointestinal problems related to cancer or its treatment.

TABLE I.6

The Management of Gastrointestinal Side Effects of Cancer Therapy

Mucositis/Stomatitis

• assess oral cavity for baseline condition and assess daily, or teach patient or family to assess daily. (See Appendix 11)

• maintain oral hygiene. Use soft toothbrush, or toothette if unable to tolerate toothbrush, after each meal; remove and clean prosthesis separately; rinse mouth after meals and at bedtime with a mild warm saline solution. If secretions are thick, or debris is difficult to remove, rinse with a sodium bicarbonate solution (one teaspoon in 500 ml of normal saline or water) every two hours.

• if mouth is dry, use fluids, atomizer mist, mouth sprays, and/or artificial saliva.

• encourage patient to avoid tobacco, alcohol, irritating foods, commercial mouthwashes, poorly fitting dentures, and lemon-glycerine swabs.

• keep lips moist with lubricating jelly.

• try soft foods, such as yogurt and cottage cheese.

• for local analgesia, try diphenhydramine hydrochloride elixir alternating with dyclonine hydrochloride or try a Maalox,diphenhydramine hydrochloride, and viscous lidocaine mixture.

Esophagitis

• try soft, creamy foods; avoid spicy foods and foods that are either very hot or very cold:

• food may need to be blenderized.

• give small frequent feedings.

• may have to be on liquid diet.

• for local anesthesia, see "mucositis/ stomatitis"; avoid aspiration due to anesthesia effect of the lidocaine.

Nausea and vomiting

• assess for fluid deficit. Monitor weight, skin turgor, urine concentration, and electrolytes.

• provide mouth care after vomiting and as needed to freshen the mouth.

• evaluate food preferences and tolerance.

• encourage small frequent feedings. Coordinate administration of antiemetics with times of eating. (See Appendix 12 for commonly used antiemetics).

• avoid fatty, spicy foods. Cold or room temperature foods are sometimes better tolerated than warm or hot foods.

• encourage clear liquids and bland foods, such as, applesauce, mashed potatoes, and toast.

• if patient is taking steroids or anti-inflammatory drugs, encourage him to take them with food.

• teach relaxation, biofeedback techniques.

• provide intravenous hydration, if necessary.

Early satiety/Cachexia/ Decreased appetite/ Taste changes

• assess circumstances of decreased intake.

• assess patient's nutritional status.

• before meals, encourage toileting, oral hygiene, pain medication, and a brief amount of exercise, if tolerated.

• encourage pleasant atmosphere and small, frequent meals which include the patient's favorite foods.

• if not contraindicated, try a small amount of sherry or wine before meals.

• encourage experimentation with spices and flavorings to enhance food flavor.

• offer nutritional supplements. Sometimes it is easier to force oneself to drink when one is not able to eat.

Constipation

• assess cause of constipation. Bowel obstruction should also be considered.

• increase bulk in the diet (bran and fresh fruit and vegetables).

• avoid cheese products.

• encourage daily fluid intake of 3,000 ml.

• assess patient's past use of laxatives.

• put patient on bowel regime and give laxative when patient has not had a bowel movement in three days.

• provide privacy for bowel movements.

• plan bowel movement for the same time each day. Give hot drink a half hour before the planned movement.

Diarrhea

• assess the patient's ability to care for himself. Encourage rest periods.

• assess for dehydration and electrolyte imbalance.

• identify source of diarrhea (i.e., treatment related, stress related).

• record character and amount of stools.

• evaluate for fecal impaction.

• avoid beverages containing caffeine.

• eliminate foods which are irritating to the GI tract, i.e., fresh fruits and vegetables, spicy food, flatus-forming food.

• encourage daily fluid intake of 3,000 ml. This may have to be increased if the diarrhea is severe.

• try frequent, low residue meals with high carbohydrate and protein intake.

• add nutmeg to food to decrease gastric motility.

• assure rectal area is cleaned carefully after each bowel movement.

• apply A & D ointment for skin protection around the anal area.

• if diarrhea is severe, recommend a liquid diet.

• administer antidiarrheal medications.

Alopecia

Although certainly not a life-threatening aspect of cancer, hair loss has a major effect on a person's self concept. Nursing can play an important role in this area by assessing the impact of alopecia on the patient and family. Teach the patient about the hair loss. Hair loss is temporary when chemotherapy is the cause; radiation therapy usually causes permanent loss of hair. Encourage the patient to cut hair short if the treatment is expected to cause alopecia.

Hair care should include the avoidance of excessive shampooing, hair dryers, sun, and exposure to the cold. The nurse can encourage the use of hats, caps, scarves, turbans, and wigs. Some health insurance plans will reimburse the cost of a wig. Wigs ahould not be used on patients receiving cranial radiation until six weeks after the completion of therapy. During radiation therapy, use of lotion for dry scalp needs to be approved by the radiation nurse or physician.

Hair loss can occur anywhere on the body. If the patient loses eyelashes, encourage the wearing of glasses. Patients should be warned that they may lose nasal hair and may have a continual "runny nose".

Programs like "Look Good, Feel Better" sponsored by the American Cancer Society encourage the patient to maintain a personal identity through the use of make-up and application of color to help minimize the changes that are occuring from treatment. Encourage the patient to maintain activities of daily living by wearing clothes that make the person feel masculine or feminine. Providing emotional support is vital in the care of the patient with alopecia.

Radiation skin reaction

Because of the development of more sophisticated radiation machines, most radiation therapy is "skin sparing" and skin reactions are not as common or as dramatic as they have been in the past. Most reactions seen today can be classified as either erythema, dry desquamation, or moist desquamation. For erythema and dry desquamation, wash the area with water only and avoid soaps. Cornstarch, baby oil, Eucerin, lanolin, A & D ointment, and Lubriderm are used to relieve the itching. Check with the radiation nurse or physician for use of specific agents.

Care of the patient with moist desquamation is controversial. Some sources suggest leaving the area open to air; others advocate covering the area with either a wet or a dry dressing. Duoderm has also been used as an alternative to a dressing. Check with the radiation nurse or physician for a preference.

ONCOLOGIC EMERGENCIES

Impending oncologic emergencies sometimes present with subtle signs and symptoms that, if detected early, may avert a crisis situation. The nurse in homecare may very well be able to assess a potentially critical situation and alert the physician before the problem becomes an oncologic emergency.

Superior vena cava syndrome

Superior vena cava (SVC) syndrome is most commonly seen in lung cancer, lymphoma, or other cancers which have metastasized to the thoracic area. Occasionally it is related to central venous catheter lines, i.e., Hickman lines.

The superior vena cava drains venous blood from the head, neck, upper extremities, and upper thorax. SVC syndrome is caused by obstruction to the blood flow; the signs and symptoms relate to the obstruction. Symptoms may develop rapidly over a one to two week period and commonly may include shortness of breath, facial swelling (with or without neck distension), swelling of trunk and arms, chest pain, cough, dysphagia, and cyanosis. Symptoms may be enhanced by lying down and therefore, may be more prominent in the morning and gradually lessen as the day progresses.

Diagnostic work-up may be deferred, depending on the rapidity of symptom build-up and the clinical picture at the time of detection. Treatment usually consists of radiation therapy to the area (although chemotherapy may be used) with a subjective response expected in about 72 hours. Diuretics may be given to provide temporary symptom relief.

Nursing interventions include:

• assess for early signs and symptoms.

• teach patient/family about reporting body changes related to SVC syndrome.

• monitor for signs of respiratory distress, provide oxygen as needed, maintain patient in Fowler's position to facilitate oxygen exchange.

• elevate arms on pillows to promote drainage.

• monitor for esophagitis/nausea from the radiation therapy.

• maintain skin integrity within the radiation field and areas of excessive engorgement.

• provide explanations and a calm environment to relieve anxiety.

Hypercalcemia

Hypercalcemia is the most common life-threatening metabolic disorder associated with cancer. It is defined as a serum calcium greater than 11 mg per 100 ml. It is associated most often with lung cancer, breast cancer, multiple myeloma, or any cancer that has metastasized to the bone. It may also be caused by hyperparathyroidism, thyrotoxicosis, prolonged and/or severe immobilization, vitamin A and D intoxication, renal failure, thiazide diuretics, and estrogens or antiestrogens used in the treatment of breast cancer. Hypercalcemia is related to excessive calcium resorption from the bone in greater levels than the kidneys can excrete.

Signs and symptoms of hypercalcemia are listed in Appendix 9.

Treatment consists of discontinuing the potentiating drugs, if applicable; hydration and diuresis to increase calcium excretion by the kidney; mobilization, if possible; drugs to inhibit bone resorption (mithramycin, calcitonin, phosphates, or glucocorticoids); dialysis, if patient has good prognosis; and chemotherapy to treat the underlying cause.

Nursing interventions include:

- monitor for signs and symptoms in high risk patients.

- teach patient/family to report changes relating to hypercalcemia.

- keep patient as mobile as possible.

- avoid dehydration. Intake should be maintained at two to three liters daily, unless contraindicated.

- assure safety if confusion exists.

- monitor for electrolyte imbalance and fluid overload/deficit secondary to hydration/diuresis therapy.

- administer specific drugs for the treatment of hypercalcemia.

Carotid artery rupture

Carotid artery rupture is an emergency that can occur in advanced head and neck cancer. The mortality rate can be as high as 60%. Exposure of the carotid artery to air, poor wound healing, previous radiation therapy to the site, previous chemotherapy, infection, poor nutritional status, and tumor growth are all contributing factors. Carotid artery rupture is a situation for which the nurse, patient, and family should be well prepared in order to avoid panic.

Nursing interventions include:

- promote wound healing by improving nutritional status, giving antibiotics as ordered, frequent dressing changes with light, non-bulky dressings, and avoidance of drying the wound.

- observe for exposure of the artery during each dressing change. Once this occurs, rupture may be imminent.

- although activity need not be restricted, have patient avoid heavy lifting or exertion, including Valsalva maneuver. Use stool softeners, if needed.

- facilitate decision making, if not done so already. It needs to be determined beforehand if the patient should be admitted to the hospital for treatment. Transfer at the time of artery rupture will most likely be in vain.

- educate the family, as digital pressure to the rupture needs to be provided immediately in order to slow bleeding and divert pulsating blood.

- have towels and sandbag available at bedside. Use to prevent the spread of blood if it cannot be otherwise controlled.

- if tracheostomy tube is in place, inflate cuff to maintain airway; insert oral airway if appropriate.

- suction blood from oral cavity or tracheostomy/ laryngectomy site.

- have syringe with previously drawn up antianxiety agent and administer.

- stay by bedside with patient.

Spinal cord compression

Spinal cord compression is caused by either metastatic tumors (especially breast, prostate, and lung) or by primary spinal cord tumors. Spinal cord compression occurs when there is invasion of the epidural space by metastasis in contiguous bone. Symptoms are related to the location of the tumor within the spinal column and can include pain, weakness, numbness and sensory loss, especially of the lower extremities, and autonomic dysfunction. Many symptoms are only vague changes in the beginning. Permanent neurologic damage can occur if not treated immediately.

Treatment most commonly consists of radiation therapy to the area of spinal cord compression, although surgical decompression is sometimes performed either alone or in conjunction with the radiation therapy. Steroids are routinely used to relieve the edema associated with spinal cord compression.

Nursing interventions include:

- explore with patient any complaint of unexplained back pain, leg weakness, constipation, difficulty voiding, or sensory loss, especially in the lower extremities.

- teach patient/family to report any body changes early.

- maintain skin integrity in radiation field and any site at risk to breakdown due to loss of mobility.

- monitor for site specific radiation side effects.

- maintain bowel and bladder function by instituting a bowel regimen and monitoring for urine retention. The patient may need intermittent catheterization or an indwelling catheter.

- if a high cervical lesion is present, may have to maintain respiratory status.

- if vertebral instability is suspected, patient may be on bedrest and/or may need to wear brace.

- administer pain medications, if needed.

- provide for safety. Patient may be at risk for injury due to unsteady gait or leg weakness.

- provide emotional support for alteration in sexual functioning, if applicable.

Brain metastasis

Patients with lung cancer (especially small cell), breast cancer, and acute leukemia are at high risk for brain metastasis. The patient may have a change in mental status or be confused. Sometimes seizures will be the presenting symptom. Treatment usually is radiation therapy, accompanied by steroids for brain edema. Surgery is sometimes performed for brain metastasis.

Nursing interventions include:

- administer intravenous hydration if the patient is comatose.

- maintain safe environment.

- reassure patient and family. The thought of getting radiation to the brain makes people fearful that they will lose control of their personality and their actions.

- provide drug teaching about steroids and anticonvulsants, if applicable.

- monitor side effects of steroids.

- if patient is started on anti-seizure medications, monitor side effects and blood levels.

- prepare patient and family for hair loss. Depending on the dose of radiation, loss may be permanent.

- monitor the scalp for skin changes.

Disseminated intravascular coagulation

Disseminated intravascular coagulation (DIC), also known as acute intravascular coagulation and consumption-coagulopathy, is a clotting abnormality most often seen in people with acute promyelocytic leukemia, although it occurs in other cancers as well. It may be either acute or chronic. DIC is characterized by both hemorrhage and uncontrolled clotting.

Symptoms include frank bleeding, petechiae, oozing from injection sites, hypotension, tachycardia, and confusion. Treatment of the underlying cause is the therapy of choice. Until DIC is controlled, transfusion of blood products are used to support the patient. Heparin may also be given but, other than in patients with leukemia, its use is controversial.

Nursing management includes early detection. Patients are usually hospitalized for acute DIC.

Home nursing management of the patient with chronic DIC includes:

- monitor for thrombus formation or bleeding.

- avoid clothing that would impair circulation.

- avoid use of "knee-gatch" on beds, "dangling" over the side of the bed, and sitting with legs in a dependent position for long periods.

- elevate the legs to encourage venous return.

- perform passive range of motion or have the patient do active range of motion exercises to the extremities.

Pericardial effusion/Cardiac tamponade

Cardiac tamponade is the impairment in circulation that occurs when the heart is compressed by pericardial fluid under pressure. It is seen in patients whose disease has infiltrated the pericardium (usually lung or breast cancer, melanoma, leukemia, or lymphoma), and in patients whose pericardium has lost its elasticity because of previous radiation to the area.

Onset may be rapid or insidious. Signs and symptoms include distension of the neck veins, pulsus paradoxus (pulse on expiration can be palpated or heard when taking a blood pressure reading, but fades on inspiration), dyspnea, hypotension, tachycardia, pericardial friction rub, chest pain and cyanosis.

Treatment usually requires hospitalization where a pericardiocentesis can be done. Mild tamponade may be treated with high dose steroids and diuretics.

Nursing interventions include:

- teach patient and family to report any changes promptly.

- place patient in Fowler's position to facilitate oxygen exchange.

- administer oxygen if needed.

- reassure patient and family, as patient may feel like he is suffocating. Remain with the patient or have someone stay with him, if possible, to ease anxiety.

Syndrome of inappropriate antidiuretic hormone secretion

Syndrome of inappropriate antidiuretic hormone (SIADH) secretion is seen in small-cell lung cancer, pancreatic cancer, Hodgkin's and non-Hodgkin's lymphoma, and thymoma, as well as in a variety of non-cancerous conditions.

Symptoms include weight gain, lethargy, weakness, nausea, irritability, and confusion. The patient has excessive fluid retention (water intoxication), is hyponatremic, and excretes large amounts of sodium in the urine.

Nursing interventions can include:

- assess for early signs and symptoms.

- teach patient and family to report body changes promptly.

- maintain fluid restriction. May be as limiting as 500 ml for a 24 hour period. Monitor intake and output.

- administer intravenous hypertonic saline (3%) solution.

- administer furosemide.

- monitor weight, urine sodium excretion, and serum electrolytes.

- maintain seizure precautions if serum sodium is less than 120.

CONCLUSION

Nursing management of the cancer patient in the home is unique. The nurse becomes the primary contact for the patient and the family. The nurse makes assessments on a regular basis. If changes in condition occurs, the nurse may be the first person to be told. This section has outlined many interventions which the nurse can use while caring for the person with cancer.

BIBLIOGRAPHY

Abernathy, E. (1987). Biotherapy: An introductory overview. *Oncology Nursing Forum, 14*(Suppl 6), 13-15.

Baird, S. (Ed.). (1991). *A Cancer Source Book for Nurses* (6th ed.). Atlanta: American Cancer Society.

Baird, S. B., McCorkle, R., & Grant, M. (Eds.). (1991). *Cancer Nursing: A Comprehensive Textbook.* Philadelphia: W.B.Saunders Co.

Baldwin, P. D. (1983). Epidural spinal cord compression secondary to metastatic disease: A review of the literature. *Cancer Nursing, 6*(6), 441-446.

Barton Burke, M., Wilkes, G. M., Berg, D., Bean, C. K., & Ingwersen, K. (1991). *Cancer Chemotherapy: A Nursing Process Approach.* Boston: Jones & Bartlett.

Brager, B. L. & Yasko, J. M. (1984). *Care of the Client Receiving Chemotherapy.* Reston, VA: Reston Publishing, Co., Inc.

Brown, M. H., Kiss, M. E., Outlaw, E. M., & Viamontes, C. M. (Eds.). (1986). *Standards of Oncology Nursing Practice.* NY: John Wiley & Sons.

Chemotherapy and You. (1990). Bethesda, MD: National Cancer Institute. (Pub. No. 91-1136).

Collins, J. L. & Thaney, K. M. (Eds.). (1988). Biotherapy: A Nursing Challenge. *Seminars in Oncology Nursing, 4* (2).

Concilus, E. M. & Bohachick, P. A. (1984). Cancer: Pericardial effusion and tamponade. *Cancer Nursing, 7*(5), 391-398.

Coward, D. D. (1986). Cancer-induced hypercalcemia. *Cancer Nursing, 9*(3), 125-132.

DeVita, V. T., Hellman, S., & Rosenberg, S. A. (Eds.). (1989). *Cancer: Principles and Practice of Oncology* (3rd ed.). Philadelphia: J. B. Lippincott Co.

Dodd, M. J. (1987). *Managing Side Effects of Chemotherapy and Radiation Therapy.* Norwalk, CT: Appleton & Lange.

Eating Hints. (1990). Bethesda, MD: National Cancer Institute. (Pub. No. 91-2079).

Groenwald, S. L., Frogge, M. H., Goodman, M., & Yarbro, C. H. (1990). *Cancer Nursing: Principles & Practice* (2nd ed.). Boston: Jones & Bartlett.

Haeuber, D. (1989). Recent advances in the management of biotherapy-related side effects: Flu-like syndrome. *Oncology Nursing Forum, 16* (Suppl. 6), 35-41.

Haeuber, D. & DiJulio, J. E. (1989). Hemopoietic colony stimulating factors: An overview. *Oncology Nursing Forum, 16* (2), 247-254.

Irwin, M. (1987). Patients receiving biological response modifiers: Overview of nursing care. *Oncology Nursing Forum, 14* (Suppl 6), 32-37.

Johnson, B. L. & Gross, J. (Eds.). (1985). *Handbook of Oncology Nursing.* NY: John Wiley & Sons.

Jones, L. A. (1987). Superior vena cava syndrome: An oncologic complication. *Seminars in Oncology Nursing, 3* (3), 211-215.

Lesage, C. (1986). Carotid artery rupture: Prediction, prevention, and preparation. *Cancer Nursing, 9* (1), 1-7.

Margolin, S. G., Breneman, J. C., Denman, D. L., LaChapelle, P., Weckbach, L., & Aron, B. S. (1990). Management of radiation-induced moist desquamation using hydrocolloid dressings. *Cancer Nursing, 13* (2), 71-80.

Morse, L. K., Heery, M. L., & Flynn, K. T. (1985). Early detection to avert the crisis of superior vena cava syndrome. *Cancer Nursing, 8* (4), 228-232.

McNally, J. C., Stair, J. C., & Somerville, E. T., (Eds.). (1985). *Guidelines for Cancer Nursing Practice.* Orlando: Grune & Stratton, Inc.

Piper, B. F., Rieger, P. T., Brophy, L., Haeuber, D., Hood, L. E., Lyver, A., & Sharp, E. (1989). Recent advances in the management of biotherapy-related side effects: Fatigue. *Oncology Nursing Forum, 16* (Suppl 6), 27-34.

Poe, C. M. & Radford, A. I. (1985). The challenge of hypercalcemia in cancer. *Oncology Nursing Forum, 12* (6), 29-34.

Radiation Therapy and You. (1990). Bethesda, MD: National Cancer Institute. (Pub. No. 90-2227).

Rooney, A. & Haviley, C. (1985). Nursing management of disseminated intravascular coagulation. *Oncology Nursing Forum, 12* (1): 15-22.

Tennenbaum, L. (1989). *Cancer Chemotherapy: A Reference Guide.* Philadelphia: W. B. Saunders.

Vetto, J., Papa, M., Lotz, M., Chang, A., & Rosenberg, S. (1987). Reduction of toxicity of IL-2 and LAK cells in humans by administration of corticosteroids. *Journal of Clinical Oncology, 5* (3), 496-503.

Wickham, R. (1989). Managing chemotherapy-related nausea and vomiting: The state of the art. *Oncology Nursing Forum, 16* (4), 563- 574.

Wood, H. A. (Ed.). (1985). Acute Complications of Cancer. *Seminars in Oncology Nursing, 1* (4).

Yasko, J. M. (1982). *Care of the Client Receiving External Radiation Therapy.* Reston, VA: Reston Publishing Co., Inc.

Yasko, J. M. (1983). *Guidelines for Cancer Care: Symptom Management.* Reston, VA: Reston Publishing Co., Inc.

CLINICAL TRIALS: INFORMATION AND OPPORTUNITIES FOR HOMECARE NURSES

Jennifer L. Guy, BS, RN, Administrator for Oncology
Park Medical Center, Columbus, Ohio 43205

CLINICAL TRIALS: INFORMATION AND OPPORTUNITIES FOR HOMECARE NURSES

Jennifer L. Guy, BS, RN, Administrator for Oncology
Park Medical Center, Columbus, Ohio 43205

INTRODUCTION

Clinical research provides the basis upon which new discoveries in biomedical science are proven to be superior to current or traditional interventions in controlling a specific disease. The clinical trial is the mechanism by which the superiority of a diagnostic or therapeutic maneuver is evaluated. Clinical research and clinical trials are conducted by applying new modalities to groups of patients meeting specific criteria, and analyzing their outcome in comparison to the known outcome of the traditional intervention in a comparable group of patients. A clinical trial can be viewed as an experiment conducted in human subjects to determine the efficacy of an intervention. (Jenkins & Hubbard, 1991) Clinical trials have traditionally been applied to therapeutic interventions; however, recently, clinical research has expanded to encompass evaluation of interventions in prevention (primary and secondary), diagnostics, symptom control, rehabilitation and palliation. (Byar & Freedman, 1990; Guy, 1991; Kessler & Sondik, 1990)

The last decade has seen dramatic changes in the delivery of health care in the United States, starting with the enactment of the Tax Equity and Fiscal Responsibility Act of 1982, and followed by almost annual legislation aimed at controlling federal spending, especially in health care. (Harris & Parente, 1991) Clearly, the site of patient care has shifted from the acute care hospital to ambulatory sites of service (physician's offices, outpatient clinics and surgical centers, skilled nursing and extended care facilities) and to the home. Increasingly sophisticated care is being provided in these alternative delivery systems, including the conduct of clinical trials.

Nurses practicing in the homecare arena can expect to become increasingly involved in the care of patients participating in clinical trials. The advent of clinical trials addressing issues in prevention, diagnostics, symptom control, and rehabilitation will require human subjects whose site of service will primarily be the home or extended care facility. Homecare, ambulatory, and extended care facility nurses will need to play an integral role in assuring appropriate conduct of these studies, and will be challenged to develop the mechanisms by which accurate data can be generated to answer clinical questions.

This chapter will emphasize cancer clinical trials, and the challenges for homecare nurses and providers. However, it is important to realize that clinical trials are conducted by all disciplines providing medical care. Homecare nurses can expect to care for clients participating in trials of antibiotics, coronary drugs, gastrointestinal agents, pain control (both drugs and devices), immune modulators, preventative interventions (behavioral/ life-style changes) and rehabilitative interventions (prostheses, exercise regimens). The principles of clinical trials apply to all modalities.

THE ORGANIZATION OF CANCER CLINICAL TRIALS

Historically, cancer clinical research has emphasized the therapeutic purview with the goal of increasing the efficacy of treatment with consideration for quality of life of the patient. Table 2.1 identifies the goals of clinical trials for persons with cancer.

TABLE 2.I

Objectives of Cancer Clinical Trials

- Improve the efficacy of treatment of malignant disease.
- Decrease the toxicity of cancer treatment.
- Improve the quality of life of the cancer patient.

Cancer clinical trials may be conducted under the auspices of the National Cancer Institute (NCI), the pharmaceutical industry, and more recently by independent research organizations. Table 2.2 illustrates the mechanisms for clinical trials as they interface with the sponsor of the clinical trials.

TABLE 2.2

Sponsors of Cancer Clinical Trials

Sponsor	Mechanism
National Cancer Institute	Clinical Cooperative Groups Cancer Centers
Pharmaceutical Industry	Selected Institutions Recruited Physician Investigators
Independent Research Groups	Collaborative Research Group of the Association of Community Cancer Centers
	National Biotherapy Study Group
	Hoosier Oncology Group

Source: Adapted from Cheson, 1991; Everson & Mannisto, 1990.

The NCI sponsored Cooperative Oncology Groups are funded by the NCI, and more recently are receiving additional funding from other groups (pharmaceutical companies, benevolent organizations). The cooperative groups consist of networks of academic institutions and community hospitals and physicians who collaborate in the design and conduct of clinical trials. Table 2.3 delineates the currently extant thirteen clinical cooperative groups, four of which are specific to pediatric oncology. Some of the cooperative groups are multimodality, addressing the gamut of malignant diseases, in all stages, and involving all modalities (surgery, radiation therapy, chemotherapy, immunotherapy); others are primary site, or disease specific, or restricted to a given modality.

Table 2.3
National Cancer Institute Cooperative Oncology Groups

Group	Modality	Population
Children's Cancer Study Group (CCSG)	multimodality	children
Pediatric Oncology Group (POG)	multimodality	children
Wilms' Tumor Study Group (NWTS)	multimodality	children
Intergroup Rhabdomyosarcoma (IRS)	multimodality	children
Gynecologic Oncology Group (GOG)	multimodality	women
Brain Tumor Cooperative Group (BTCG)	multimodality	brain tumor patients
National Surgical Adjuvant Breast and Bowel Project (NSABP)	multimodality	adjuvant therapy in breast and bowel cancers in adults
Radiation Therapy Oncology Group (RTOG)	radiation therapy	radiation sensitive tumors
Cancer and Leukemia Group B (CALGB)	multimodality	adults
Eastern Cooperative Oncology Group (ECOG)	multimodality	adults
European Organization for Research and Treatment of Cancer (EORTC)		
North Central Cancer Treatment Group (NCCTG)	multimodality	adults
Southwest Oncology Group (SWOG)	multimodality	adults

NCI designated comprehensive cancer centers also sponsor clinical trials in oncology for patient participation, as well as participate in the cooperative group clinical research efforts. An NCI designated comprehensive cancer center is generally an academic institution that receives funding from NCI, based on meeting eight criteria important to the care of the cancer patient. (Cheson, 1991). Often, the clinical trials emanating from the centers are the pilot studies on which the larger cooperative group studies are based. Comprehensive cancer centers are also obligated to conduct laboratory research, epidemiological studies, education (public and professional), and community outreach programs.

The mechanisms by which physicians may participate in clinical trials, and thus, offer participation to their patients occurs in several ways. Each mechanism has established criteria and credentials review upon which participating physicians and institutions are selected to participate in clinical cancer research, all aimed at ensuring safe implementation of the clinical trial that will generate valid scientific data to answer the clinical question. In the 1970's, it became apparent that as more medical, surgical, and radiation oncologists were practicing in the community, clinical trials had to be disseminated to theses sites , as opposed to being limited to the university setting to enable wider patient participation, and thus, more rapid completion of the studies. The NCI has four programs which allow access to clinical trials to physicians and patients in the community. These are outlined in Table 2.4.

TABLE 2.4

NCI Sponsored Community Clinical Research Programs

Mechanism	Participants	Focus	Source of Trials
Cooperative Group Outreach Program (CGOP)*	Community physicians & institutions	Treatment	Cooperative group (1)
Community Clinical Oncology Program (CCOP)**	Community physicians & institutions	Treatment Cancer Control	>1 research base, cooperative group/center
Minority Community Clinical Oncology Program (Minority CCOP)**	Community physicians & institutions serving minority populations	Treatment Cancer Control	>1 research base, cooperative group/center
High Priority Clinical Trials Program**	Community physicians & institutions	Treatment	Phase III cooperative group trials in common cancers***

*Affiliation with academic cooperative group member required.
**Independent relationship with research bases.
***Designated Trials selected by Cooperative Group Chairman: studies require large numbers of patients, and are expected to answer important questions in common malignancies.

Source: Adapted from Cheson, B. D. (1991). Clinical trials program. Seminars in Oncology Nursing, 7 (4), 235-242.

The pharmaceutical and biotechnology industry has long been instrumental in conducting clinical research in malignant disease. This has been accomplished both by collaboration with the NCI, and by independently recruiting qualified physicians to conduct trials of new agents in their institutions. Pharmaceutical trials provide the basis on which new agents can come to market, and provide the necessary data for a New Drug Application (NDA) to the Food and Drug Administration. The last decade has resulted in an explosion in the development of new agents with potential efficacy in the treatment of malignant disease, especially in the area of biological products. Because of the large numbers of new agents, the need for increasing numbers of qualified clinical investigators to conduct studies of the efficacy of these agents rapidly has become acute. Simultaneously, the constraints in funding experienced at the federal level have inhibited timely evaluation of these new agents. Thus, independent research groups are developing to recruit investigators and their patients into clinical trials evaluating the role of new agents in the treatment of cancer, the control of toxicities, and in palliation. Among such efforts are the Collaborative Research Group of the Association of Community Cancer Centers which acts as a liaison between its members and national pharmaceutical and biotechnology companies to further community based clinical investigation of new cancer therapy products (Everson & Mannisto, 1990). These types of efforts will, hopefully, improve the speed with which the efficacy of new interventions can be determined. Other independent research efforts extant restrict themselves to specific modalities, or issues in cancer patient care.

Table 2.5
TYPES OF CANCER CLINICAL TRIALS

Treatment	Cancer Control
Phase I: First trials in humans; establish dose, establish toxicity; define pharmacology of the agent	Prevention: risk identification /risk reduction, mechanisms of inducing lifestyle change to decrease risk
Phase II: Determine efficacy in specific malignancy; confirm/ expand phase I data	Screening: motivating screening, validating methods
Phase III: Compare new therapy to the standard therapy; evaluate diagnostic methods; compare improvement in cure/control, toxicities, quality of life	Diagnosis/Detection: evaluating diagnostic methods (imaging, laboratory test) and techniques Treatment: compliance
Phase IV: Elicit more information about the drug once it has been released for commercial use. Determine the principles for combined modality and the associated problems	Quality of Life Issues: methods of alleviating/minimizing toxicity (drugs, behavioral, scheduling, nutrition, fatigue, etc) Rehabilitation: methods/interventions to maximize/expedite (exercise, prostheses, surgical procedures) rehabilitation; survivorship Terminal Care: pain control, evaluate spiritual, and psychosocial interventions, test bereavement interventions

TYPES OF CANCER CLINICAL TRIALS

Cancer clinical trials can be divided into two broad categories: therapeutic (treatment) trials and cancer control trials. Table 2.5 outlines the two categories and their emphasis.

The types of clinical trials are not mutually exclusive. Often, a cancer control study may be incorporated into a therapeutic protocol as a collaborative-companion study, which is conducted in concert with the medical treatment protocol. Collaborative companion studies address issues in the management of side effects of the treatment under study, or the relative quality of life of subjects receiving protocol therapies. Parallel companion studies are those that address nursing issues generated by a medical intervention or treatment protocol. (Farrell & Cohen, 1991)

The Clinical Protocol

The document that outlines a clinical trial is the protocol. (Melink & Whitacre, 1991) Both therapeutic and cancer control trials follow a defined research plan which consists of the components illustrated in Table 2.6.

TABLE 2.6

Major Components of a Clinical Trial

Objectives:	the clinical question the study addresses
Background:	the scientific data that justifies the trial, and establishes the clinical question as requiring evaluation
Patient Eligibility:	defines the patient population to be included in the study; consent requirements
Intervention:	defines the trials intervention and how it is to be implemented
Evaluation Criteria:	standardized criteria for evaluating response to the study intervention, determining toxicities, calculating survival, or detecting a difference between groups
Statistical Evaluation:	the statistical methods used to analyze the data obtained
Data Management:	how the data will be collected, collated, and presented for analysis

The methodology of a clinical trial depends on the type of trial and the endpoint of the study. Treatment trials generally determine response rate, duration of response, and survival. Cancer control trials will emphasize different endpoints, such as a decrease in the incidence or severity of toxicity, prevention of an adverse effect, superiority of quality of life, or improved functioning.

Clinical trials emanating from the cooperative groups and pharmaceutical industry undergo vigorous scrutiny for scientific validity by numerous committees, and approval bodies with specific expertise in the area under study prior to their accrual of patients to the trial. All clinical trials, by law, must be reviewed by an Institutional Review Board (IRB) who is charged with the protection of human subjects. The composition of the IRB is defined by law. The IRB must review the study for its ethical conduct, scientific validity, and risk/benefit ratios for the subjects to whom participation will be offered. The IRB assures that human subjects are enrolled only after their informed consent is given, in writing. The consent must include: identification of the investigational nature of the study, the purpose of the study, a description of the procedures to which the patient will be subjected, as well as the safeguards incorporated into the intervention to minimize adverse effects. The potential risks and benefits, as well as costs, alternatives to the protocol-proposed intervention, compensation, rights to emergency treatment, designation of individuals (by name and telephone access) from whom additional information can be obtained, and voluntary participation (or refusal/ withdrawal rights) without compromise of additional care are also required to be included in the consent form. The consent document must also include parameters for the protection of patient confidentiality, by defining to whom patient records may be made available for review. Only after IRB approval, which then requires yearly re-review of the study until its conclusion, and informed consent has been obtained, can the clinical trials intervention proceed. (DHHS, 1981)

IMPLEMENTATION OF CLINICAL TRIALS: ISSUES FOR HOMECARE

With the shift of cancer care to the outpatient arena, homecare nurses are increasingly caring for patients participating in clinical trials, both in the direct provision of protocol therapy, and in the monitoring of patients receiving new therapies. For home care nurses, and oncology nurses this presents some exciting new challenges.

Table 2.7 defines potential issues the home care nurse may be asked to address when caring for clients participating in clinical trials.

TABLE 2.7

Clinical Trials Issues for the Homecare Nurse

Issue	Nursing Implications
Recruitment	a) Identify patients eligible for clinical trials
	b) Assessment of compliance potential with the proposed intervention
	c) Confirmation of eligibility, i.e. performance status, by direct observation in the home setting
	d) Patient education regarding clinical trials
Consent	a) Interpreting the consent form for patients
	b) Assisting patients to obtain adequate information to consent to participate
Implementation	a) Provision of the protocol required intervention i.e., providing direct care and treatment
	b) Monitoring for toxicity
	c) Assessing compliance
	d) Obtaining and documenting clinical data
	e) Observing and reporting response to the study interventions
Long Term Followup	a) Identifying and reporting long term toxicities
	b) Reporting long term patient outcomes
Clinical Trials in Home Care	a) Designing and conducting clinical trials in home care of the cancer patient

Timely and adequate recruitment to clinical trials participation is a major issue in advancing cancer care. Currently it is estimated that only 10 to 30% of patients eligible for a cancer clinical trial actually participate in one (Wittes & Friedman, 1988). Homecare nurses are in an ideal position to educate the client on the benefits of clinical trials participation as state of the art care, and thus, foster accrual to protocols.

By developing mechanisms to implement protocol care at home, a new cadre of patients may be available for recruitment to protocol participation. To do so requires that the homecare nurses become knowledgeable about the clinical trials participation of physicians and institutions that refer patients to their agency. Mechanisms must be devised for the administration of protocol therapies at home, such as specialized training in the administration of chemotherapy, and biologics, or the performance of protocol interventions such as relaxation techniques, or the direction of rehabilitative efforts. Systems must be developed and policies and procedures written for the control of investigational agents, obtaining study required laboratory tests, and reporting their results, assessing response and toxicity according to protocol specific criteria, and providing documentation of same to the clinical investigator conducting the study. Home care nurses are in the best position to observe and document performance status when observing patients at home, an evaluation parameter of all clinical trials which has been difficult to accurately assess in a weekly visit to the office or clinic, or while the patient is hospitalized.

In some malignancies, continuous infusion chemotherapy has been investigated, and some data exists that it may be superior to intermittent bolus therapy. However, implementation of definitive clinical trials has been difficult due to the requirement for use of portable infusion pumps, and supervision in the home. From this perspective, homecare nurses provide the vital link for evaluation of this hypothesis by managing patient therapy at home.

The role of growth factors, used as adjuncts to antineoplastic therapy, are being defined in clinical trials. Because many are self-administered, the homecare nurse will often be assisting patients in their administration. Appropriate administration teaching, and observation of toxicities are imperative to establish their efficacy in cancer treatment. Homecare nursing observations of compliance, toxicity, and response are invaluable.

In cancer control research, the homecare nurse is in the unique position to assess, and foster patient compliance with protocol treatment. It is anticipated that many of these studies will encompass lifestyle changes. Nurses observing patients in their home environment will make valuable contributions in reinforcing the desired behavior, and in making observations of compliance.

Motivating clients to obtain cancer screening examinations is another role for the home care nurse, and an area of research that presents fertile ground for initiation via the homecare agency, who can best identify barriers to effective implementation of such initiatives.

CLINICAL RESEARCH OPPORTUNITIES FOR HOMECARE NURSES

Research opportunities exist to define the role of home nursing care and its effect on quality of life of the cancer patient. McCorkle, et al (1989), conducted a study of home nursing care as compared to intermittent office care in patients with lung cancer. This study showed a positive impact on symptom distress in the homecare group, but a negative impact on health perceptions compared to the office care group. Additional research is needed to best define the implications of these findings.

As the economics of medical care in the United States change, with an emphasis on controlling costs, clinical trials will be forced to address issues related to the cost/benefit ratios of cancer patient care. Studies documenting the cost-effective aspects of delivering cancer patient care in the home, applying prevention strategies, and utilizing screening and early detection methodologies, and home based palliative and rehabilitative interventions will become increasingly important. Homecare providers must start to address these issues by conducting clinical research in the homecare populations that they serve, and must scientifically validate their impact on the quality of care, the cost effectiveness of their services, and the outcome of their care.

REFERENCES

Byar, D.P., Freedman, L.S. (1991). The importance and nature of cancer prevention trials. *Semin Oncol 17*:413-424.

Cheson, B.D. (1991). Clinical trials programs. *Semin Oncol Nurs 7*:4, 235-242.

Department of Health and Human Services (1981). *Protection of Human Subjects:* Informed Consent. Washington, DC, Federal Register, January 27, part IX.

Everson, L.K., Mannisto, M.M. (1990). ACCC's collaborative research group: an update. *Oncol Issues 5*:4, 15.

Ferrell, B.R., Cohen, M.Z. (1991). Companion studies. *Semin Oncol Nurs 7*:4, 253-259.

Guy, J.L. (1991). New challenges for nurses in clinical trials. *Semin Oncol Nurs 7*:4, 297-303.

Harris, M.D., Parente, C.A. (1991). Home care services, in Baird, S.B., McCorkle, R., Grant, M., (eds). Cancer Nursing: *A Comprehensive Textbook*. Philadelphia, PA, Saunders, pp 1023-1032.

Jenkins, J., Hubbard, S. (1991). History of clinical trials. *Semin Oncol Nurs 7*:4, 228-234.

Kessler, L.G., Sondik, E.J. (1990). Achieving a public health impact from cancer control research. *Semin Oncol 17*:495-503.

McCorkle, R., Benoliel, J.Q., Donaldson, G., Georgiadou, F., Moinpour, C., Goodell, B. (1989). A randomized clinical trial of home nursing care for lung cancer patients. *Cancer, 64*:6, 1375-1382.

Melink, T.J., Whitacre, M.Y. (1991). Planning and implementing clinical trials. *Semin Oncol Nurs 7*:4, 243-251.

Wittes, R.E., Friedman, M.A. (1988). Accrual to clinical trials. *JNCI 80*:12, 884-885.

SUGGESTED BIBLIOGRAPHY

Garvey, E.C. (1987). Current and future nursing issues in the home administration of chemotherapy. *Semin Oncol Nurs 3*:2, 142-147.

Kessler, D.A. (1989). The regulation of investigational drugs. *N Engl J Med 320*:5, 281-288.

Ochs, J., Mulhern, R., Kun, L. (1988). Quality of life assessment in cancer patients. *Am J Clin Oncol* (CCT) *11*:3, 415-421.

Passamani, E.(1991). Clinical trials — are they ethical? *N Engl J Med 234*:22, 1589-1591.

Szunyog, C.L. (1989). Coordinated home care: the vital link. *NITA*, November/December, 491-494.

Varricchio, C.G., Jassak, P.F. (1989). Informed consent: an overview. *Semin Oncol Nurs 5*:2, 95-98.

BONE MARROW TRANSPLANTATION: A HOMECARE PERSPECTIVE

Kevin Sowers, MSN, RN
Oncology Clinical Nurse Specialist
Duke University Medical Center, Durham, N.C.

Mary Ann Crouch, MSN, RN Head Nurse
Adult Bone Marrow Transplant Unit
Duke University Medical Center, Durham, N. C.

BONE MARROW TRANSPLANTATION: A HOMECARE PERSPECTIVE

Kevin Sowers, MSN, RN
Oncology Clinical Nurse Specialist
Duke University Medical Center, Durham, N.C.

Mary Ann Crouch, MSN, RN Head Nurse
Adult Bone Marrow Transplant Unit
Duke University Medical Center, Durham, N. C.

In 1992, the United States will witness a 12% increase in persons diagnosed with cancer since 1987 (American Cancer Society, 1992). This increase will continue to expedite the exploration of advancements being made in medical, biotechnological and genetic engineering over the next decade.

Historically, the development and study of new cancer therapies has improved the prognosis of many fatal neoplasms. Bone marrow transplantation (BMT) is one such therapy that was formerly a highly experimental and rarely used procedure, but has now become a more common and accepted treatment for many malignant and non-malignant disorders.

HISTORICAL PERSPECTIVE

BMT was historically used only as a salvage therapy for advanced diseases, but now with the technological advancements and increased awareness of the need for supportive care measures, patients are enjoying extended disease-free survivals. Table 3.1 is a brief summary of the evolution of bone marrow transplantation:

TABLE 3.1

Historical Evolution of BMT

Date	BMT Procedure
1891	Bone marrow used as an oral nutritional treatment for patients with anemia.
1930	Intramedullary and intravenous infusions of marrow used to treat patients with anemia.
1940	Study of marrow failure with the discovery of atomic energy.
1950	High dose chemoirradiation and marrow grafts studies, involving persons with end-stage leukemia. Studies then stalled until 1960s related to the lethal antigen-antibody immunologic reaction of the bone marrow graft versus host.
1960	Advent of human histocompatibility typing, blood product pheresis, and effective antibiotic therapies for the treatment of infections unlocked BMT as a viable treatment for malignant and non-malignant disorders.
1980s	Outpatient care of post-transplantation patients.

Source: Adapted from Santos, G. (1983). History of bone marrow transplantation. Clinical Hematology, 12, 611-639.

BMT has been established as an effective experimental treatment for selected patient populations, with more than 10,000 transplants having been performed worldwide (Cooper, 1984). The International Bone Marrow Transplant Registry reveals that the median age of BMT recipients is 20 years, with one half of all transplants having been performed on children. BMT was pioneered with children, with the first successful allogeneic BMT performed by Good and colleagues on a 5 month old boy with severe combined immunodeficiency syndrome (Gatti, 1968).

TYPES OF BONE MARROW TRANSPLANT

The type of transplant a patient receives will be dependent upon the source of the marrow. There are three sources of donor marrow: allogeneic, autologous, and syngeneic.

Allogeneic

This method refers to marrow taken from a human leukocyte antigen (HLA) matched sibling. In theory, the donor could be related or unrelated to the patient, but at this time only HLA-matched siblings are used. There are documented cases of allogeneic transplants between individuals who were only partially HLA-matched, but a higher incidence of graft rejection is noted in these individuals (Appelbaum, 1988; Dinsmore, 1982). Allogeneic is the most common type of BMT presently being used in the United States.

Autologous

Autologous BMT is often used in patients with malignancies that are at high risk for relapse. This method employs the use of the patient's own marrow. Relapse is a possibility for patients receiving autologous BMT. It is uncertain whether the etiology of this relapse is the result of a reinfusion of tumor cells or the failure of the chemoirradiation treatment. (Buchsel, 1990).

Syngeneic

This method uses stem cells obtained from an identical twin donor. A higher incidence of relapse is reported in syngeneic transplants secondary to what appears to be an antileukemic effect of graft-versus-host disease (Applebaum, 1981).

DISEASES TREATED WITH BONE MARROW TRANSPLANTATION

Malignant and non-malignant disorders are the two categories of diseases treated with bone marrow transplants in adults and children (see Table 3.2). BMT research is ongoing, with the results creating new pathways for future therapies and techniques. This research will broaden the application and utilization of this treatment regime in the next decade (Thomas, 1982).

49

TABLE 3.2

Diseases Treated with Bone Marrow Transplantation

Malignant Diseases

Autologous	Allogeneic	Syngeneic
Leukemia	**Leukemia**	**Leukemia**
Refractory	Acute Myelocytic	Acute Myelocytic
	Acute Lymphocytic	Acute Lymphocytic
	Chronic Myelocytic	Chronic Myelocytic
		Hairy Cell
Lymphoma	**Lymphoma**	**Lymphoma**
Burkitt's	Non-Hodgkin's	Non-Hodgkin's
Undifferentiated		
Diffuse Histiocytic		
Melanoma		**Sarcoma**
		Ewing's
Sarcoma		
Soft tissue		
Ewing's		
Rhabdomyosarcoma		
Solid Tumors		
Breast		
Lung		
Ovary		
Testis		

Non-malignant Diseases

Aplastic Anemia	Lipidosis
Chronic Granulomatous	Mucopolysaccharidosis
Combined Immunodeficiency Disorders	Osteopetrosis
Diamond-Blackfan Syndrome	Reticular Dysgenesis
DiGeorge's Syndrome	Sickle Cell Anemia
Fanconi's Anemia	Wiskott-Aldrich
Gaucher's Disease	Syndrome

PHASES OF BONE MARROW TRANSPLANT

Bone marrow transplant protocols may vary from cancer setting to cancer setting, but the basic BMT process is similar.

Pre-transplant evaluation

The span between diagnosis and BMT treatment will be dependent upon the individual's diagnosis and condition, and the treatment priorities at the cancer setting. Newly diagnosed patients with anemia may be treated within hours of their diagnosis, unlike the leukemic population which may receive transplant years after diagnosis.

An extensive patient and family assessment is performed on each potential BMT candidate. This assessment explores the patient's medical history, a physical exam, and an individual and family psychological and spiritual evaluation. In allogeneic transplant human leukocytic antigen (HLA) typing is performed on family members during this time.

Once the patient meets the criteria established for admission, donor selection is the next step in the BMT process. The most appropriate type of BMT is based upon three factors (Freedman, 1990): (1) the disease or disorder, (2) availability of HLA donors, and (3) health status of potential donors.

A tour of the BMT facilities pre-transplant is often helpful for patients and families, because fear of the unknown is often common during this phase. Introducing the BMT environment, answering questions and beginning patient/family teaching has been beneficial as a component of the pre-admission procedure. Patients may also have a bone marrow harvest and central venous access device placed during this time.

Bone marrow harvesting

The patient in autologous transplant or donor for allogeneic transplant is taken to the operating room (OR) to have his/her bone marrow harvested. Marrow is aspirated from the posterior and/or anterior iliac crest. The amount of bone marrow aspirated is dependent upon the body size of the patient (Child-300 cc; Adult-800-1000 cc.). The marrow is then heparinized to prevent clotting. Further processing of the bone marrow may be required, such as cryopreservation, pharmacologic and immunologic purging, and t-cell depletion. Special processing will depend upon the transplant center's protocol, and may vary between allogeneic and autologous transplant recipients.

Nursing care after bone marrow harvest encompasses monitoring for signs and symptoms of bleeding, infection and pain at the harvest site. Patients should be encouraged to be up and ambulating once the effects of general anesthesia are no longer present.

Conditioning

Conditioning is the extended hospitalized phase in BMT designed to eradicate the patient's original marrow and residual tumor cells with high-dose chemotherapy and/or total body irradiation (TBI). Researchers are currently focusing on the dosing, timing, and sequencing of the chemotherapy and TBI to assure the best tumor kill with the least toxicities.

Nursing care during this phase involves accurate administration of chemotherapy and monitoring for potential side effects. Side effects will be discussed in the post infusion/engraftment section. The patient and family require consistent emotional support and accurate, timely answers concerning therapy and progress.

Treatment Environment

The conditioning treatment leaves the person receiving the BMT open to opportunistic infections secondary to the depletion of white blood cells and the alteration in the immune response. This is one of the leading causes of death in the post-transplant patient. Therefore, BMT teams will elect to implement many of the following protective measures: (1) room isolation procedures with laminar air-flow systems, (2) gut decontamination with nonabsorbable oral antibiotics and low bacteria diet, (3) prophylactic antibiotic administration for *Pneumocystis carinii* and herpes virus.

Bone Marrow Transplant Treatment Modalities

Bone marrow transplantation, unlike standard therapies, has made it possible to administer chemotherapy and/or radiotherapy in lethal doses in order to kill a higher percentage of tumor cells. Table 3.3 lists the majority of the chemotherapy agents used in BMT and the potential side effects.

TABLE 3.3

Chemotherapy Agents Used in Bone Marrow Transplantation

Chemotherapy	Short-term Side Effects	Long-term Side Effects
BCNU (Carmustine, BiCNU)	Severe hypotension Facial flushing Chest pain Myelosuppression Nausea/vomiting Stinging at infusion site Low grade fever Dizziness Ataxia	Gynecomastia Headache Neuroretinitis Fibrosis/dyspnea Tachypnea Rales Decreased Breath sounds BUN elevation
Busulfan (Myleran)	Myelosuppression Transient LFTs Hyperuricemia Hyperuricosuria	Adrenal Insufficiency Gynecomastia Testicular atrophy Impotence Amenorrhea Teratogenic effects Hyperpigmentation Alopecia Cataracts Interstitial pulmonary fibrosis

(continued)

Chemotherapy	Short-term Side Effects	Long-term Side Effects
CCNU (Lomustine, CeeNU)	Nausea/vomiting Diarrhea Stomatitis Myelosuppression Transient LFTs Lethargy	Anorexia Alopecia Renal failure
Cisplatin (CDDP, Platinol)	Nausea/vomiting Diarrhea Transient LFTs Rare anaphylaxis Hypokalemia Hypomagnesemia Hypocalcemia Hyperuricemia Nephrotoxicity	Anorexia Alopecia High frequency hearing loss Tinnitus Color vision loss Peripheral neuropathy Papilloedema Retrobulbar neuritis Nephrotoxicity
Cytarabine(Cytosine Arabinoside, Ara-C, Cytosar-U)	Nausea/vomiting Diarrhea Mucositis Stomatitis Abdominal pain Myelosuppression Transient LFTs Conjunctivitis Skin rashes Cellulitis at infusion site	Thrombophlebitis Anorexia Cerebellar toxicity Slurred speech Ataxia Staggered gait
Cytoxan (Cyclophosphamide, Neosar, CTX)	Acute hemorrhagic Voltage on EKG Tachycardia CHF SOB Hypotension JVD SIADH Nausea/vomiting Mucositis Hemorrhagic cystitis Headache	Anorexia Bladder carcinomas Dysplasia Amenorrhea Azoospermia Teratogenicity Testicular atrophy Alopecia Interstitial pneumonitis Metallic taste Myelosuppression
Daunorubicin (DNR, Cerubidine, Caunomycin HCL, Rubidomycin HCL)	Nausea/vomiting Diarrhea Mucositis Red urine Myelosuppression Alopecia Fever	Congestive heart failure Arrhythmias Impotency

Chemotherapy	Short-term Side Effects	Long-term Side Effects
Dibromodulcitol (DBD, Mitolactol, Elobromol)	Nausea/vomiting Diarrhea Myelosuppression Vertigo Somnolence Visual hallucinations Tumor pain Dyspnea	Anorexia Hyperpigmentation BUN
Doxorubicin (Adriamycin-PFS, Adriamycin-RDF, Hydroxydaunorubicin HCL, Hydroxudaunomycin HCL)	Nausea/vomiting Mucositis Stomatitis Diarrhea Red urine Myelosuppression Anaphylaxis	Arrhythmias Pericarditis Cardiomyopathy Congestive heart failure Impotency
Etoposide (VP-16, VePesid)	Hypotension Nausea/vomiting Diarrhea Myelosuppression Erythema Headache Bronchospasm Fever/chills Anaphylaxis	Pancreatitis Paresthesia Mucositis
Melphalan (L-PAM, Alkeran)	Nausea/vomiting Diarrhea Stomatitis Myelosuppression Proteinuria BUN/Creatinine Hypotension Diaphoresis Cardiac arrest	Myelodysplastic syndromes Acute Leukemia Dermatitis Fibrosis

(continued)

Chemotherapy	Short-term Side Effects	Long-term Side Effects
PCNU (Piperidylnitrosourea)	Hypotension Nausea/vomiting Stomatitis Myelosuppression Seizures	Anorexia
Thiotepa (Thio-TEPA)	Nausea/vomiting Stomatitis Myelosuppression Headache Dizziness Altered mental status Hives Bronchoconstriction	Anorexia Peripheral nerve damage Demyelination Paresthesia
Thioguanine (6-TG,2-Amino-6--mercaptopurine)	Nausea/vomiting Stomatitis Diarrhea Myelosuppression Rash Hyperuricemia	Anorexia Hepatic vein occlusion Photosensitivity Loss of vibration sensitivity Unsteady gait

Bone marrow infusion

The re-infusion time of the marrow will be dependent upon the treatment center's protocol. Autologous marrow is frozen and brought to the unit on "day zero", or better known as the nadir of the conditioning phase. The marrow is then thawed to body temperature and infused via the central venous access device.

Bone marrow reinfusion should be handled similarly to a red blood cell transfusion. Patients may be pre-medicated to prevent reactions such as fever and chilling. Hard candy or lemon drops may be helpful in preventing nausea and vomiting related to marrow preservative. Other potential side effects may include pulmonary embolus, cardiac arrhythmias, anaphylaxis and hyper/hypotension. It is important to monitor cardiac rhythm and vital signs pre-, during and post-marrow re-infusion.

Postinfusion/Engraftment period

The infused bone marrow usually requires 14 days to regenerate. The literature reflects that autologous marrow recovery rates are slower than those observed for allogeneic and syngeneic transplants. Many feel that this is secondary to autologous bone marrow being frozen and the fact that the bone marrow is taken from individuals who have received drugs which cause granulocytopenia (Cogliano-Shutta, 1985). A patient may take as long as one year to regain normal immune function.

Buchsel (1990) describes the theory of BMT as simple in concept, but difficult to implement related to the toxicities associated with high-dose chemotherapy and irradiation. The complications occurring after BMT can be interrelated and categorized as acute or chronic. Acute complications are those appearing beyond day 100 of transplant (Ford, 1988). Further discussion of this postinfusion/engraftment period includes a systems approach to acute treatment related toxicities, brief medical management and nursing care. Chronic complications will be discussed in the discharge phase.

ACUTE COMPLICATIONS

Neuromuscular Complications

The patient undergoing BMT is at risk for many potential neurologic complications. Complications can be related to high-dose conditioning regimens, irradiation, infective processes, as well as supportive therapies initiated post transplant.

Common chemotherapeutic agents used during the transplant process may cause neurologic toxicity. These agents may include carmustine, etoposide, cytosine arabinoside (ara-c) and cisplatin. Ara-c is commonly used as an agent to treat leukemia and the side effects include: headache, somnulence, personality changes, memory loss, confusion, and slurred speech. These intense neurologic effects are due to Ara-c's long half life in cerebrospinal fluid. Ara-c in high doses may cause cerebellar dysfunction manifested as ataxia, dysarthria, nystagmus, and muscle weakness (Bolwell, et al. 1988).

Other potential neurologic events include peripheral neuropathies, color vision changes, and high frequency hearing loss. These are commonly caused by the drug cisplatin, which is frequently used for the autologous transplant of solid tumors. Irradiation used in a conditioning regimen may cause fatigue, weakness, and confusion.

Infections that may effect the neurologic status of a patient undergoing BMT may be bacterial, fungal, or of viral nature. The patient undergoing BMT, as an uncompromised host, is susceptible via many portals of entry. Fungal infections with aspergillus species account for 50-57% of central nervous system infections in these patients. Viral infections usually involve cytomegalovirus and varicella-zoster (Davis and Patchell 1988). Drugs used to prevent or decrease severity of effects of graft versus host disease (GVHD) may also cause neurologic changes (see Table 3.4).

TABLE 3.4

Drugs Used for GVHD Prophylaxis and Treatment

Drug	Potential Side Effects
Cyclosporine	tremors, seizures, confusion,
Methotrexate	paresthesias, weakness, coma,
Steroids	somnolence, fatigue, agitation,
Antithymocyte globulin and OKT-3	psychosis, increased intracranial pressure, pressure

The focus of medical and nursing care of neurologic effects is prevention and early detection. Maintaining isolation techniques to assure a clean environment to prevent infection, and monitoring side effects of drug administration are important nursing interventions. If neurologic toxicity occurs, patient safety issues become a major focus of care.

Cardiac
Cardiac complications seem to occur most commonly in the autologous transplant population as opposed to the allogeneic population. Table 3.5 represents identified risk factors for the development of cardiac toxicity.

TABLE 3.5

Identified Cardiac Toxicity Risk Factors

1. Prior therapy with anthracyclines
2. Chest radiotherapy
3. Cyclophosphamide dose greater than 150mg/kg
4. Cyclophosphamide and TBI as transplant conditioning
5. Sepsis
6. Mitral Valve disease
7. Ejection fraction of less than 50%

Adapted from Whedon, M. B. (1991). Bone Marrow Transplantation: Principles, Practices, and Nursing Insights.Boston: Jones & Bartlett, p. 198.

In therapies prior to BMT, many patients receive anthracyclines such as doxorubicin. This predisposes the patient to cardiac failure (von Herby, et al. 1988). Characteristic damage by anthracyclines as a group includes: cellular degeneration, destruction of myocardial fibrils and mitochondrial changes. Symptoms exhibited by patients may include peripheral edema, tachycardia, dyspnea, and rales (Wilke, 1991).

Cyclophosphamide in high doses causes hemorraghic myocardial necrosis accompanied with pericardial effusions. This toxicity occurs within days of cyclophosphamide therapy. Patients often exhibit signs of congestive failure, cardiomegaly, and peripheral edema. Of particular interest is the decrease in voltage on EKG.

When severe, hemorraghic myocarditis may cause cardiac tamponade and lead to subsequent death. Treatment for tamponade includes: intravenous fluid management, vasopressive therapy, and often pericardiocentesis. The transfusion of platelets post cyclophosphamide therapy may play a role in prevention of hemorraghic myocarditis. In a study conducted by Panella (1990), platelet function was noted to be abnormal during and after high-dose cyclophosphamide therapy. The administration of platelets post therapy improved platelet function.

Cardiac damage may result when a patient has had previous chest irradiation. Damage may involve development of pericardial effusions, and constrictive pericarditis. Patients undergoing transplant with a history of chest irradiation may have their heart shielded to prevent any potential injury. (Wilke, 1991).

Cardiac infections may occur during the transplant process. They are rare. Pathogens that may cause infection include: aspergillus, candida albicans, pseudomonas, clostridium, streptococcus, coxsackie virus, and adenovirus (Sale & Shulman, 1984).

Pulmonary

Interstitial pneumonitis is the most common pulmonary toxicity associated with allogeneic transplantation. Bortin (1983) describes three predisposing factors: an immunosuppressed host, lung damage, and presence of opportunistic microorganisms. Any or all of the predisposing factors can have an effect on the development of pneumonitis. Generally, peak incidence of interstitial pneumonitis is two months after transplant and will be discussed in the discharge phase.

The autologous transplant population also experiences a toxic pulmonary effect, usually with the same symptoms noted above. Generally, the disorder is not related to infection, it is related to latent effect of high-dose carmustine therapy. The result is pulmonary fibrosis, often requiring intubation and ventilatory support. In addition, steroid therapy is initiated and generally an open lung biopsy is performed.

Gastrointestinal

Common gastrointestinal side effects that patients may experience include: (a) nausea and vomiting, (b) mucositis, and (c) veno-occlusive disease. Nausea and vomiting occurs as a direct result of high-dose chemotherapy and TBI as well as other supportive therapies such as antibiotics and immunosuppressants used to prevent GVHD. Nausea and vomiting is an individual experience, as patients experience varying degrees from mild to severe. This may result in electrolyte disturbances as well as nutritional deficits increasing the need to monitor the patients' nutritional status (Vanacek, 1991). In addition, patients may experience anorexia, and taste changes. It is not uncommon for patients to require parenteral nutrition during this hospitalized phase.

Many antiemetics are used to control nausea and vomiting. Clinical trials are underway to test combinations of antiemetics in BMT patients (Vanacek and Gilbert, 1989). Nursing's role is to monitor nausea and vomiting and treat as medically prescribed. Other interventions that may benefit the patient include relaxation therapies and providing a quiet, calm environment.

Mucositis is a side effect of preparative transplant regimens (Carl and Higby, 1985); the entire gastrointestinal tract is at risk. Mucositis occurs as a result of injury to epithelial tissue. Oral mucositis occurs early after conditioning and generally resolves when marrow engrafts. Oral mucositis can be extremely painful requiring parenteral narcotics for relief. Patients may experience dysphagia and be unable to eat food. Meticulous mouth care is vital; many regimens incorporate frequent use of normal saline or bicarbonate solutions as rinses. Oral antifungal agents along with systemic antibiotics, antifungal and antiviral agents may be used to prevent and/or treat infections of the oral cavity.

Diarrhea occurs as a form of mucositis. It may be one of the first indications of graft versus host disease. Diarrhea may cause the patient to experience abdominal cramping and pain. Bleeding and infection may occur as complications from diarrhea. Treatment of diarrhea includes: (a) identifying and treating the underlying cause, (b) controlling any fluid and electrolyte imbalances that may result, (c) providing symptomatic relief for the patient, and (d) protecting skin in the rectal area from breakdown. Opioid drugs may commonly be used to control diarrhea. Caution must be used especially when an infective organism may be present. Strict assessment of volume status and the monitoring and replacement of fluid and electrolytes are imperative nursing measures in caring for patients with diarrhea. Meticulous rectal care should be performed routinely after each episode of diarrhea, keeping the rectal area clean and dry. Ointments may be used as moisture barriers. If and when breakdown does occur, the patient is at a risk for developing infection. Infection may be bacterial, fungal, viral, or protozoal. Appropriate drug therapies for treatment should be maintained (Vanacek, 1991).

Veno-occlusive Disease

Sinusoids in the liver that become occluded by collagen or reticulum fibers cause veno-occlusive disease. Obstruction of the sinusoids causes back flow of blood, thus causing fluid to drain into the lymphatics. This fluid eventually flows to the peritoneal cavity causing ascites. Clinically, patients experience sudden weight gain, right upper quadrant pain, ascites, jaundice, hepatomegaly, and encephalopathy.

Twenty one percent of bone marrow transplant patients experience veno-occlusive disease (VOD). About half of these cases are self limiting and spontaneously resolve. The other half die as a result of VOD. Factors that predispose bone marrow patients to VOD include: high-dose chemotherapy and radiation therapy as conditioning regimens, liver abnormalities, leukemia, allogeneic versus autologous transplant, and age greater than 15 (Jones, et al, 1987; McDonald, et al, 1985).

Nursing management of the patient with VOD is complex and challenging. Many of these patients become critically ill and require nursing staff specially trained in intensive care. Management incorporates maintaining fluid and electrolyte balance and renal integrity; avoiding coagulopathy and encephalopathy; and minimizing the effects of ascites while assuring appropriate redistribution of body fluids (Ballard, 1991).

Genitourinary

Renal insufficiency and failure may occur as a result of BMT. Numerous etiologies may contribute to renal complications. Chemotherapy used for conditioning may cause acute damage to the tubules in the kidney. Cisplatin is one example of an agent whose dose limiting toxicity is nephrotoxicity.

Hemorraghic cystitis is a transplant complication that occurs with high-dose cyclophosphamide therapy. Acrolein, a metabolite of cyclophos-phamide, causes ulceration of the bladder mucosa, resulting in hemor-rhage into the bladder (Sale and Shulman, 1984). Bleeding may be life threatening in the severe form and painful obstruction can develop with blood clot formation in the bladder. Treatment of hemorrhagic cysitits begins with prevention. Three noted interventions have proven beneficial in the prevention of hemorrhagic cystitis. These include: (a) vigorous irrigation of the bladder with sterile saline (100 cc-1000 cc) during and for twenty-four hours post administration of cyclophosphamide; (b) vigorous intravenous hydration; and (c) concurrent mesna and cyclophos-phamide administration (mesna binds with acrolein preventing bladder damage). If hemorrhagic cystitis occurs, treatment includes vigorous bladder irrigation and platelet transfusions to arrest bleeding. Cystoscopy, with cauterization of ulcerated areas may be required to stop bleeding (Ballard, 1991).

Rapid tumor lysis due to chemotherapy may also cause renal damage in lymphoma and leukemia patients. This syndrome is characterized by hyperuricemia, hyperkalemia, hyperphosphatemia, and hypocalcemia. Precipitation of uric acid and phosphate in renal tubules may result in acute renal failure (Lydon 1986).

Supportive drug therapies used to treat transplant side effects may also cause renal damage. Some of the drugs include: amphotericin-B, aminogylcosides, dopamine, levophed, cyclosporine, and methotrexate.

Hypovolemic states, induced by sepsis, hemorrhage, veno-occlusive disease and dehydration, may prevent adequate renal perfusion, potentially causing damage to the kidneys. Nursing care includes assessment of renal status. This includes monitoring blood chemistries and drug levels, safe and accurate administration of nephrotoxic drugs, and maintaining fluid and electrolyte balance.

Hematopoietic/Immunologic

Profound neutropenia occurs as a result of high-dose chemotherapy and TBI regimens. Neutropenia usually lasts for two to four weeks following transplant. Despite recovery of white cell count, normal immune function may not return for months after transplant (Atkinson, 1990). This period of neutropenia and decreased immune function places a transplant patient at risk for development of infection. The most common pre-engraftment infections include: gram negative and gram positive bacteremias, fungal sepsis and herpes simplex infection. Early post engraftment, BMT patients are susceptible to cytomegalovirus, fungi, gram positive organisms, and *Pneumocystis carinii* (Wingard, 1990). Interventions to protect BMT patients from acquiring infections include: isolation in laminar air flow environment, high efficiency particulate air (HEPA) filtration, and reverse isolation. BMT patients are often restricted to low bacterial count diets, and must drink sterile water. Patients may be placed on prophylactic oral antibiotics to suppress normal flora that could become pathogens (Pizzo, 1989). Febrile episodes are immediately treated with intravenous broad spectrum antibiotics, providing coverage for both gram positive and gram negative organisms. Antifungal coverage is often added when a patient remains febrile three or more days after initiation of broad spectrum antibiotics. Patients generally continue with bacterial and fungal coverage until they experience adequate neutrophil recovery.

Nursing interventions include protecting the patient from potential infective organisms. This begins with adherence to protective isolation techniques. Frequent assessment should occur for early detection of infection. Strict hygienic regimens, such as, meticulous oral and perianal care, should be initiated and use of central venous access devices (VAD) should incorporate sterile technique.

BMT patients also experience anemia and thrombocytopenia as a result of therapy. Patients receive frequent transfusions of red blood cells and platelets. To prevent side effects, such as fever and rigors, patients may be pre-medicated with tylenol and benadryl. Blood products are irradiated to kill donor t-lymphocytes. Blood products which are seronegative for cytomegalovirus (CMV) are often used to prevent the development of CMV infections. Platelet recovery can be delayed in some BMT patients and may require measures to prevent and protect the patient from bleeding should be implemented.

Acute Graft Versus Host Disease

Graft versus host disease (GVHD) occurs when donor t-lymphocytes reject the host — the patient undergoing transplant (Wagner, Vogelsang, and Beschorner, 1989). GVHD primarily occurs in allogeneic transplant patients (40-50%) but has been reported in the autologous patient population (Hood, et al. 1987). Clinical manifestations involve the skin, liver, and gastrointestinal tract. Acute GVHD occurs within the first one hundred days post transplant.

The skin exhibits the first signs of acute GVHD. A maculopapular rash spreads over the palms, soles, and ears. Bullae, ulcerations, and necrosis may occur, resulting in epithelial desquamation. With liver involvement there is hepatomegaly, right upper quadrant pain, an increase in bilirubin, alkaline phosphatase, and SGOT levels. Liver failure may occur, resulting in green, watery diarrhea and abdominal cramping that may progress to sloughing of intestinal mucosa.

Therapies to prevent and treat GVHD have been developed. Single agent or combination therapies with the following drugs are common: methotrexate, corticosteroids, cyclosporine and antithymocyte globulin. Nonpharmacologic techniques include: t-lymphocyte depletion from donor marrow prior to transplant by using agglutination techniques, immunoadsorption columns, and treatment with monoclonal antibodies.

Care of the patient with the graft failure is supportive, as death due to infection or hemorrhage is likely. Nursing management of acute GVHD includes assessment of skin integrity, gastrointestinal function and hepatic function. Meticulous skin care to prevent infection and promote comfort is important. Use of creams to prevent dryness, medications to treat pruritus, and special beds, may be necessary. Monitoring of intake and output, and electrolyte status is also important because, severe diarrhea and mucosal sloughing may lead to malabsorption resulting in nutritional deficits and electrolyte imbalances. Parenteral hyperalimentation may be required if malabsorption occurs. Monitoring for occult blood may detect early gastrointestinal bleeding. Hepatic function should be monitored by laboratory data related to the increased incidence of encephalopathy and bleeding with liver dysfunction.

Psychosocial

The BMT patient has many concerns during the period of hospitalization. These may include: coping with side effects (nausea/vomiting), prolonged hospitalization and isolation, and impact of the BMT on the family.

Physical symptoms can be very stressful for a BMT patient. Research has concluded that there are relationships between psychological variables and severity of symptoms such as pain, nausea and vomiting. Beneficial therapies to control symptoms include use of behavioral techniques such as hypnosis, relaxation training, and biofeedback (Ahles and Shedd, 1991).

Prolonged hospitalization and confinement to protective isolation may be a stressor to the BMT patient. Although rationale for protective isolation is understood, patients may exhibit anxiety, depression and feelings of powerlessness and helplessness. A nursing intervention would be to give the patient as much control as possible over care and routines. The nurse must provide a supportive atmosphere for the patient to freely express concerns and needs. Body image concerns such as alopecia, weight loss, and fear of major treatment related toxicities are of concern. For a patient not experiencing toxicities, boredom prevails. It is appropriate to provide diversional activities such as recreational therapy, physical therapy, and visits from family and volunteer staff.

The family of the BMT patient plays a vital role in the recovery of the patient. It is important for many families to become involved in the care of the patient. Families often feel helpless during hospitalization. Providing information about progress and teaching strategies which assist the patient in activities of daily living (ADL) may help decrease the feelings of helplessness. A shift in family roles may also occur when family members are placed in situations that they are unaccustomed to. This "role reversal" may be stressful for a spouse who feels uncomfortable or overwhelmed with his/her new responsibilities.

The nurse should be aware of the concerns of the patient and family during the transplant process. Nursing can provide reassurance and support; consultation of mental health professionals helps the family adjust to the transplant process.

Psychosocial care of the pediatric patient should incorporate knowledge of normal growth and develoment with age specific interventions. Table 3.6 illustrates developmental issues of pediatric BMT patients.

TABLE 3.6

Concerns of Pediatric Transplant Patients

Age	Concern	Interventions
Infant	Separation Anxiety	Encourage parent to perform ADL's
	Fear of Strangers	Provide consistency with staff and routines
		Provide age appropriate toys
Toddlers	Separation Anxiety	Limit separations from parents, incorporate parents into care
	Loss of Control	Limit separation from parents, incorporate parents into care
Preschool	Body Injury	Establish as much routine as possible
	Loss of Control	Explain procedures in simple terms, use play techniques
	Fear of the Unknown	Have parents bring child's favorite blanket, toys
School Age	Bodily Harm	Have child participate in self care
	Loss of Control	Involve parents in care routines
	Death	Provide school tutor
	Negative Feeling About Self	Provide activities such as video games, crafts, schoolwork
Adolescent	Altered Body Image	Encourage friends to call and visit
	Lack of Privacy	Explain procedures and answer questions
	Decreased Independence	Allow patient to decorate room
	Feeling Different from Peers	Provide diversional activities such as: television, music, reading, video games

The health care team must establish trust with the family and patient. Care should include a team approach, with a family centered focus. Not uncommon are the parents' feelings of anger, fear, helplessness, and a sense of loss of control. Parents may feel guilty about the sick child and the lack of time necessary for other children in the family. Incorporating parents into daily care, helping manage day to day crisis, and providing an open atmosphere for parents to express their feelings are all nursing interventions. Healthy siblings may feel neglected and resentful. The nurse should encourage parents to openly communicate with their children; siblings should be allowed to visit; attendance at support sessions that may be available for the family are ways to intervene with the family. The sibling who is the marrow donor should be provided with updates on the progress of their sibling; the donor often feels left out during transplant recovery (Abramovitz, 1991).

CHRONIC COMPLICATIONS

Discharge/ Homecare

Patients surviving BMT may be "disease free", but develop chronic complications secondary to the treatment. The survival rates after treatment are dependent upon (1) the age of patient (> 30 risk for GVHD, interstitial pneumonia, VOD of the liver), and (2) the remission and clinical status of the patient at the time of transplant (Cheson, 1986). Young children appear to be more resilient to organ system failure than adult BMT populations. High-dose chemotherapy and radiation can be devastating to children, related to increased metabolic rate, developing organs and the lack of effective coping responses to deal with the stress of transplantation.

Patients will be discharged from treatment centers based on discharge criteria. This discharge criteria often focuses on: (1) the ability to take nutrition, fluids, and medication by mouth, (2) the treatment and/or disease symptoms controlled with medications, (3) afebrile status, (4) stable blood counts and (5) the availability of people, resources and support in the home.

With the advent of growth stimulating factors, bone marrow transplant patients are being discharged earlier in their engraftment period. The post-BMT patient in the home setting should be monitored and evaluated at regular intervals for early detection and treatment of acute and chronic complications. The chronic complications associated with BMT will be explored through a body system approach.

Neuromuscular

Patients receiving cranial or spinal irradiation combined with intrathecal chemotherapy prior to high-dose conditioning have reported leukoencephalopathy (generalized necrosis of the white matter of the brain), myasthenia gravis, and cognitive dysfunction.

Chronic neuromuscular effects can also be attributed to treatment of GVHD (graft versus host disease). TBI and long-term steroid therapy for graft versus host disease (GVHD), can lead to the development of cataracts. Peak time for cataract formation is 3-6 years after BMT. Patients may have corrective surgery with lens implants or contact lenses. Hypomagnesemia causing seizure activity in marrow recipients taking cyclosporine for chronic GVHD has also been described.

Pulmonary

Restrictive and obstructive pulmonary lung disease is observed in approximately 10-13% of patients post transplant. Pulmonary status can range from mild to severe pulmonary insufficiency, but often improves with time. Interstitial pneumonia occurs in 10-20% of long term survivors and carries a 50% mortality rate (Sullivan, 1986). Specific type of pneumonia include idiopathic, CMV, varicella zoster virus and *Pneumocystis carinii* pneumonia. The peak incidence for this is two months post BMT. Instituting prophylactic antibiotic therapy for patients at risk for interstitial pneumonia has resulted in decreased incidence of late pneumonia. A potential source for pulmonary infections may be related to the sinusitis that occurs secondary to dryness of the upper airway and sinus membranes post BMT.

Cardiac

Chronic cardiac complications are rare and related to the chemotherapy/radiation administered during the conditioning phase. Constrictive pericarditis may result from radiation therapy to thoracic cavity or from specific chemotherapy agents. This complication may lead to the development of congestive heart failure.

Gastrointestinal

Gastrointestinal symptoms are related to GVHD and are discussed in the hematological section.

Genitourinary

Chronic renal failure may be a complication encountered by persons who have developed renal toxicities secondary to the administration of high-dose chemotherapy, cyclosporine, and amphotericin B (Cade, 1987). Dialysis may be a component of the long-term treatment plan.

Integumentary

The integumentary system is effected by GVHD and is discussed in the hematological section.

Hematopoietic/Immunological

GVHD can affect 25-50 % of the patients living more than 100 days after an allogeneic BMT (Deeg, 1984). Chronic GVHD resembles an autoimmune disease, and may affect the skin, musculoskeletal system, eyes, mouth and GI tract. Table 3.7 outlines the clinical presentation of chronic GVHD.

TABLE 3.7

Clinical Presentation of Chronic GVHD Post-BMT

Body Organ	Clinical Presentation
Skin	**Initial:** • Dryness • Hyperpigmentation/ hypopigmentation • Maculopapular erythematous rash • Hair loss • Nail ridging **If untreated may lead to:** • Scleroderma • Contractures
Musculoskeletal	• Muscle weakness • Muscle pain • Decreased range of motion
Ocular	**Initial:** • Burning • Grittiness • Dryness • Photophobia **If untreated may lead to:** • Keratoconjunctivitis sicca • Cornea wasting
Oral	• Intraoral lesions • Decreased keratinization • Decreased saliva production • Increased risk of dental caries
Esophageal	• Pain and difficulty in swallowing
Gastrointestinal	• Steatorrhea • Nausea/vomiting • Weight loss/Anorexia • Diarrhea
Liver	• Liver enzymes • Hepatomegaly • RUQ pain
Infections	• Bacterial and fungal infections

This complication may also cause damage to the lacrimal and salivary glands. Treatment for GVHD include: cyclosporine, cortiocosteroids, azathioprine, and experimental studies with monoclonal antibodies and thalidomide.

Skin changes are usually the first presentation of GVHD. The maculopapular erythematous rash may present on the patient's trunk, palms, soles, and ears. If the skin conditions go untreated, chronic GVHD may progress to scleroderma and contractures (Press, 1987). Interventions for the alterations occurring to the skin include: antipyretics, application of lanolin based creams and <1% hydrocortisone cream, and use of natural soaps and lotions without perfume to prevent further dryness. Persons should also be advised to avoid sun exposure without protection.

GVHD musculoskeletal complications may be characterized by muscle weakness and/or pain with decreased range of motion. Steroids used for the treatment of GVHD may put patients at risk for aseptic necrosis and associated joint pain.

The incidence of ocular involvement with chronic GVHD is 80-90%. (Thomas, 1975). Patients may begin by stating that they have burning and grittiness in their eyes, which is caused by a decrease in tear production. Photophobia may also occur and is felt to be caused by corneal changes (Sullivan, 1985). Management revolves around the use of artificial tears and corticosteroids. Lacri–Lube™ ophthalmic ointment may be applied at bed time to prevent the eyes from drying out during sleep. Protective eyewear or "patching" is also recommended to prevent the evaporation of moisture in the eyes. The patient should be followed by an ophthalmologist.

Eighty percent (80%) of the patients with chronic GVHD have some type of oral involvement. Intra-oral lesions, reduced keratinization, and decreased saliva flow due to oral sicca may be present. Dental hygiene should be taught since there is increased risk for dental caries. Weight loss may occur due to inadequate nutritional intake. Ongoing nutritional assessments are imperative in patients experiencing clinical manifestations of GVHD to the mouth, esophagus, and gastrointestinal tract.

Esophageal complications associated with chronic GVHD can also lead to decreased oral intake and weight loss. Patients presenting with pain and difficulty in swallowing usually have a diagnostic work-up including a barium swallow and endoscopic exam with a culture and biopsy. Esophageal dilatation may be required.

Chronic GVHD effects on the gastrointestinal tract can be experienced by 25-35% of the patients with GVHD. The signs and symptoms can include steatorrhea, nausea and vomiting, diarrhea and weight loss. Anorexia can become a long-term complication in this population. The BMT team should rule out a fat malabsorption syndrome if the patient has persistent diarrhea. A GI series with a small bowel follow through, stool cultures and endoscopy are usually in order to rule out gastrointestinal infections. Hyperalimentation and rest for the GI tract are interventions if patients are experiencing weight loss and/or fluid and electrolyte imbalances.

The liver is affected in 90% of the patients presenting with GVHD (McDonald, 1986). Elevated liver enzymes, hepatomegaly, and RUQ pain are the first signs of GVHD liver involvement. A screen for hepatitis, abdominal ultrasound to rule out obstruction, and a liver biopsy to rule out infection are often the diagnostics used in the interpretation of these clinical symptoms.

Chronic GVHD increases incidence of late infections secondary to B and T cell deficiency (Lum, 1981). Bacterial infections of the lungs, sinuses, and blood are most frequently seen secondary to the patient's inability to manufacture functional immunoglobulins. Prophylactic antibiotic regimes are often implemented to avoid the presentation of late infections.

Post-BMT patients should avoid contact with persons who may have the chicken pox virus as they are susceptible to varicella zoster virus (VZV). Varicella zoster is the virus responsible for chicken pox and shingles. Studies reveal that 30-35% of patients develop VZV by one year post-BMT (Locksley, 1985). Patients may present with fever, chills, unexplained persistent pain and itching prior to the development of vesicles. VZV can be life-threatening if it goes untreated. Medical intervention usually consists of the implementation of IV acyclovir. If the patient knows that they have had contact with someone with chicken pox, a varicella zoster immune globulin (VZIG) injection can be administered. The VZIG injection must be given within 96 hours after exposure. Severe pain along the tract of the nerve may be present for weeks after the VZV vesicles have resolved.

One year after BMT, the patient should have immune function tests performed. The results of the skin tests will mandate the plan for the immunizations needed. Pneumovax, influenza, polio, diptheria, pertussis and tetanus toxoid are several of the booster vaccines usually recommended. Live virus vaccines should be avoided.

Endocrine

Effects on the endocrine system are dependent on age of the patient, dose, and duration of the treatment. The problems encountered with the endocrine system, post-transplant, can be divided into those involving the thyroid, gonad, or growth hormone.

General malaise, decreased endurance, and delayed growth patterns in children are related to the dysfunction of the thyroid. Children conditioned with high-dose chemotherapy alone have normal growth and development, but the inclusion of TBI may cause abnormalities of growth rates in children (Corcoran - Buchsel, 1986). Children may experience low self esteem secondary to delayed growth patterns and should receive appropriate psychological interventions.

Hormonal replacement that includes estrogen and progesterone is necessary for long-term relief in postpubertal females who are symptomatic (see Appendix 13, Table 8). Alterations in the vaginal vault may result in painful intercourse, making vaginal dilators and estrogen cream necessary for stenosis of the vagina.

Psychosocial

The psychological and spiritual ramifications of the post-BMT phase impact every aspect of the patient and family's life. Rehabilitation and re-entry into society become a major focus of the discharge plan of care (see Appendix 13, Table 9).

The most common emotions experienced by patients and family are guilt, relief, anger, depression, anxiety, and fear. The patient's and family's ability to respond to these emotions will be based upon their developmental stage, educational level, prior history with stressful events, the use of effective coping strategies in the past, and the patient's health status.

The quality of life of persons surviving BMT will vary depending on the presence and severity of long-term complications. The post-BMT patient may be "cured", but still dealing with chronic illnesses. Quality of life and survivorship issues need further exploration as the post-BMT patient's life span increases.

Secondary malignancy and relapse

The long-term complication of secondary malignancies may be attributed to several variables such as: high-dose chemotherapy and TBI, long-term immunosuppressive therapy, Epstein-Barr syndrome, or residual tumor cells not eradicated by the conditioning protocol (Deeg, 1984). Documentation of an increased incidence of secondary malignancies may be related to the increased life span of persons post-BMT. Instruction in self-breast and testicular exams are imperative because of the risk of second malignancy development.

Relapse of leukemia remains a concern despite the advancements being made in BMT. Harboring host-cells untouched by the chemotherapy and/or radiation are often the etiology of this complication. Success in the treatment of BMT relapses is limited, but the patient may choose to explore additional treatment options or may choose no further interventions.

FUTURE TRENDS

The future of BMT is exciting, but additional research is necessary to further develop more effective combinations of chemotherapeutic agents and irradiation techniques. Advances in these treatment modalities will decrease the incidence of relapse post BMT. More technological advances for the detection, prevention and treatment of graft-versus-host disease are necessary. Trials continue to investigate how antibiotics are used to treat infections associated with transplantation.

Marrow purging techniques will continue to be developed. Currently, trials using monoclonal antibodies bound to magnetic spheres are being used to "purge" a patient's marrow to decrease risk of marrow contamination with tumor. Purging marrow with pharmacologic agents such as 4-hydroxycyclophosphamide (4-HC) and mercocyanine are currently under investigation.

Technologic advances with peripheral blood stem cells may also have an impact on BMT. Peripheral stem cells are removed from BMT patients before the conditioning phase by leukopheresis. They are cryopreserved like bone marrow. When thawed and reinfused, peripheral stem cells repopulate in the bone marrow; a remanufacturing of blood components occurs. This advancement may replace the need for surgical harvesting of bone marrow.

Biologic response modifiers such as G-CSF (granulocyte colony stimulating factor) and GM-CSF (granulocyte-macrophage colony stimulating factor) are currently used in investigations to enhance function and stimulate early recovery of white blood cells. In some cases (especially with autologous BMT), colony stimulating factors have decreased the period of neutropenia and number of infections experienced by BMT patients (Peters, 1989). Future trials may describe enhanced roles of biological response modifiers.

Genetic disorders may be treated in the future by gene transfer. In this process defective material may be replaced by healthy genetic material. Gene transfer has been successful in a laboratory setting and may have future implications for BMT (Thomas, 1987).

Economics

Support for a transplant program within an institution requires extensive support from many services. The American Society of Clinical Oncologists (1991) recommends special commitment from organizations involved in allogeneic and autologous transplant. Criteria include: (a) a supportive patient volume with at least 15-20 bone marrow transplants per year, (b) appropriate facilities, including a unit with 2 or more designed transplant beds; equipment necessary for marrow processing and cryopreservation; air-handling systems and supplies for protective isolation; and 24 hour radiology and laboratory resources, (c) qualified personnel, including BMT trained physicians, nurses, social workers and subspecialty physicians available for consultation; ancillary services with a commitment to transplant, (d) treatment outcomes demonstrating sufficient numbers of patients treated in a focused disease group, and (e) data reporting that is timely, accurate and communicated to appropriate registries and medical literature.

It is not surprising, to comply with the above criteria, BMT becomes an expensive procedure. Average cost of BMT has been reported as $75,000-200,000 (Welch & Larson, 1989; Reed, 1991). Additional expenses for BMT may include: (a) processing of donor marrow, (b) pre-admission work-up, (c) labs and scans, (d) right atrial catheter insertion, (e) supplies for care as well as travel related costs incurred (Bedell, 1991).

Insurance reimbursement for BMT varies; common allogeneic transplant for leukemia receives third party reimbursement, but it is less likely that autologous transplant for solid tumors will. It is through the refinement of therapy and technique that issues of reimbursement will lessen.

The effort to decrease costs may impact on reimbursement of transplant procedures. Future development of outpatient related facilities for transplant will be developed (Peters, 1991). Long term visionary planning for outpatient BMT services will be needed as we enter this next decade of cancer care.

BIBLIOGRAPHY

Abramovich, L. (1991). Perspectives on pediatric bone marrow transplantation. In M. B. Whedon (Ed.), *Bone marrow transplantation: Principles, practice and nursing insights* (pp. 70-104). Boston: Jones and Bartlett.

Ahles, T. & Shedd, P. (1991). Psychosocial impact of bone marrow transplantation in adult patients: Prehospitalization and hospitalization phases. In M. B. Whedon (Ed.), *Bone marrow transplantation: Principles, practice and nursing insights* (pp. 280-292). Boston: Jones & Bartlett.

American Cancer Society, (1992). Facts and figures. *CA: A cancer journal for clinicians.* Atlanta: American Cancer Society.

American Society of Clinical Oncologists (1991). Recommended criteria for the performance of bone marrow transplantation. In E. Brown (Ed.), *Proceedings of the DATTA forum on high dose chemotherapy and autologous hematopoietic support as a treatment of breast cancer* (pp. 35-36). Chicago: American Medical Association.

Appelbaum, R., Fefer, A., Cheever, M., et. al. (1981). Treatment of non-Hodgkin's lymphoma with marrow transplantation in identical twins. *Blood, 58,* 509.

Appelbaum, F. (1988). Bone marrow transplantation. In R. Wittes (Ed.), *Manual of oncologic therapeutics.* Philadelphia: J. B. Lippincott Co.

Atkinson, K. (1990). Reconstruction of the haemopoietic and immune systems after transplantation. *B. M. T., 5,* 209-226.

Ballard, B. (1991). Renal and hepatic complications. In M. B. Whedon (Ed.), *Bone marrow transplantation: Principles, practice, and nursing insights* (pp. 362-377). Boston: Jones & Bartlett.

Bedell, M. (1991). Procedure cost and reimbursement issues. In M.B. Whedon (Ed.), *Bone marrow transplantation: Principles, practice, and nursing insights* (pp. 362-377). Boston: Jones & Bartlett.

Bortin, M. M. (1983). Pathogenesis of interstitial pneumonitis following allogeneic bone marrow transplantation for acute leukemia. In R.P. Gale (Ed.), *Recent advances in transplantation.* (pp. 445-460). New York: Alan R. Liss.

Bowell, B. J. et. al. (1988). High-dose cytarabine: A review. *Leukemia,* 2, 253-260.

Buchsel, P. (1990). Bone marrow transplantation. In S. Groenwald, M. Frogge, M. Goodman, & and C. Yarbro, (Eds.), *Cancer nursing: Principles and practice* (2nd ed.), (pp. 307-337). Boston: Jones & Bartlett.

Buckner, A., et. al. (1984). Pulmonary complications of marrow transplantation. *Experimental Hematology* (suppl 15), *12,* 1-5.

Cade, R., Wagemaker, H., Vogel, S., et. al. (1987). Hepatorenal syndrome studies of the effect of vascular volume and intraperitoneal pressure on renal and hepatic function. *American Journal of Medicine, 39,* 427-437.

Carl, W. & Higby, D. J. (1985). Oral manifestations of bone marrow transplantation. *American Journal of Clinical Oncology, 8,* 81-87.

Caudell, K. A. (1991). Graft-versus-host disease. In M. B. Whedon (Ed.), *Bone marrow transplantation: Principles, practice, and nursing insights* (pp.160-181) Boston:Jones & Bartlett.

Cheson, B., Curt, G., (1986). Bone marrow transplantation: Current perspectives and future directions. *Journal of National Cancer Institute, 76,* 1265-1267.

Cogliano-Shutta, N., Broda, E., & Gress, J. (1985). Bone marrow transplantation: An overview and comparison of autologous, syngeneic, and allogeneic treatment modalities. *Nursing Clinics of North America, 20,* (1), 49-65.

Corcoran-Buchsel, P. (1986). Long-term complications of allogeneic bone marrow transplantation: Nursing implications. *Oncology Nursing Forum, 13,* 61-70.

Davis, D. & Patchell, R. A. (1988). Neurologic complications of bone marrow transplantation. *Neurology Clinics, 6,*377-387.

Deeg, J., Storb, R., Thomas, E. (1984). Bone marrow transplantation: A review of delayed complications. *British Journal of Haematology, 57*(2), 185- 208.

Deeg, J., Sanders, J., Marin, P., et.al. (1984). Secondary malignancies after marrow transplantation. *Experimental Hematology, 12,*660-666.

Deeg, H.J., et.al. (1988). *A guide to bone marrow transplantation.* New York: Springer-Verlag.

Deisseroth, A., Abrams, R., Holohan, R., et. al. (1982). Blood component replacement applications of the continuous flow centrifuge, and bone marrow transplantation. In A. Levie (Ed.), *Cancer in the young* (pp. 285-298). New York: Masson Publishing USA, Inc.

Dinsmore, R., & O'Reilly, R., (1982). Bone marrow transplantation: Current status. *Pathobiology Annual, 12,* 213-231.

Duke University Medical Center Bone Marrow Transplant Staff (1991). *Standards of Nursing Care for Allogeneic and Autologous Bone Marrow Transplant.* Durham: Duke University.

Ford, R., Ballard, B., (1988). Acute complications after bone marrow transplant. *Seminars in Oncology Nursing, 4,*15-24.

Freedman, S., Shivnan, J., Tilles, J., & Klemm, P., (1990). Bone marrow transplantation: Overview and nursing implications. *Critical Care Nursing, 13,* (2), 51-62.

Gatti, R., Menwissen, H., Allen, H., et. al. (1968). Immunological constitution of sex-linked lymphopenic immunological deficiencies. *Lancet, 2,* 1366-1369.

Hood A. F., (1987). Acute graft-versus-host disease: development following autologous and syngeneic bone marrow transplantation. *Archives of Dermatology, 123,*: 745-750.

Jones, R. J., et. al. (1987). Veno-occlusive disease of the liver following bone marrow transplantation. *Transplantation, 44* (6), 778-783.

Locksley, R., Flournoy, N., Sullivan, K., et. al. (1985). Infection with varicella-zoster virus after marrow transplantation. *Journal of Infectious Disease, 152,* 1172-1181.

Lum, L., Seigneuret, M., Storb, R., et. al. (1981). *In vitro* regulation of immunoglobulin synthesis after marrow transplantation. *Blood, 58,* 431-439.

Lydon, J. (1986). Nephrotoxicity of cancer treatment. *Oncology Nursing Forum, 13* (2), 68-77.

McDonald, G. B., et. al. (1985). The clinical course of 53 patients with veno-occlusive disease of the liver after marrow transplantation. *Transplantation, 39* (6), 603-608.

McDonald, G., Shulman, H., Sullivan, K., et. al. (1986). Intestinal and hepatic complications of human bone marrow transplantation. *Gastroenterology, 90,* 460-477.

Panella, T. (1990). Platelets acquire a secretion defect following high-dose chemotherapy. *Cancer, 65,* 1711-1716.

Peters, W. P. (1989). The effect of recombinant human colony-stimulating factors on hematopoietic reconstitution following autologous bone marrow transplantation. *Seminars in Hematology, 26,* 18-23.

Peters, W. P. (1991). Personal communication. Outpatient transplants for breast cancer.

Pizzo, P. A. (1989). Considerations for the prevention of infectious complications in patients with cancer. *Reviews of Infectious Diseases, 11* (Supplement 7), 1551-1563.

Press, O., Schaller, R., Thomas, E. (1987). Bone marrow transplant complications. In L. Toledo-Pereyra (ed.) *Complications of organ transplantation,* (pp. 399-424). New York: Marcel Dekker.

Reed, E. (1991). The ABMT itself: Intensity of resources. In E. Brown (Ed.)., *Proceedings of the DATTA forum on high dose chemotherapy and autologous hematopoietic support as a treatment of breast cancer* (pp. 35-36). Chicago: American Medical Association.

Sanders, J., Pritchard, S., Mahoney,P., et. al. (1986). Growth and development following marrow transplantation for leukemia. *Blood, 68,* 1129-1135.

Santos, G., (1983). History of bone marrow transplantation. *Clinical Haematology, 12,* 611-639.

Sullivan, K. (1985). Special care of the allogeneic marrow transplant patient. In P. Wiernik, G. Canellos, R. Kyle, C. Schiffer (Eds.), *Neoplastic diseases of the blood* (pp. 117-1140). New York: Churchill Livingstone.

Sullivan, K., Meyers, K., Flournoy, N., et. al. (1986). Early and late interstitial pneumonia following human bone marrow transplantation. *International Journal of Cell Cloning, 4* (supplement), 107-121.

Thomas, E., Storb, R., Clift, R., Fefer, A., et. al. (1975). Bone marrow transplantation. *New England Journal of Medicine, 292,*(16), 832-843, 895-902.

Thomas, E. (1982). Bone marrow transplantation: Present status and future expectations. In K. Isselbacher, R. Adams, E. Braunwald, et. al. (Eds.), *Harrison's principles of internal medicine* (pp. 135-152). New York: McGraw-Hill.

Thomas, E. (1987). Bone marrow transplantation to the year 2000. In R. P. Gale & R. Champlin (Eds.), *Progress in bone marrow transplantation UCLA symposium on molecular and cellular biology new series, 53* (pp. 905-910). New York: Alan R. Liss.

Thompson, C., June, C., Sullivan, K., et. al. (1984). Association between cyclosporine neurotoxicity and hypomagnesemia. *Lancet, 2,* 1116-1120.

Vanacek, K. (1991). Gastrointestinal complications of bone marrow transplantation. In M. B. Whedon (Ed.), *Bone marrow transplantation: Principles, practice,and nursing insights* (pp. 206-239). Boston: Jones & Bartlett.

Vanacek, K. & Gilbert, C. (1989). A randomized, double blind antiemetic study in autologous bone marrow transplant patients. *Oncology Nursing Society* (in progress).

van der Wal, R., Nims, J., Davies, B. (1988). Bone marrow transplantation in children: Nursing management of late effects. *Cancer Nursing, 11*(3), 132-143.

von Herbay, A., et. al. (1988). Cardiac damage in autologous bone marrow transplantation in acute nonlymphocytic leukemia. *New England Journal of Medicine, 321*(12), 801-812.

Wagner, J., Vogelsang, G., & Beschorner, W. (1989). Pathogenesis and pathology of graft-versus-host disease. *AJPHO, 11*(2): 196-212.

Welch, H. G. & Larson, E. B. (1989). Cost-effectiveness of bone marrow transplantation in acute nonlymphocytic leukemia. *New England Journal of Medicine, 321*(12), 807-812.

Wikle, T. J. (1991). Pulmonary and cardiac complications of bone marrow transplantation. In M. B. Whedon (Ed.), *Bone marrow transplantation: Principles, practice and nursing insights* (pp. 182-205). Boston: Jones & Bartlett.

Wingard, J. (1990). Management of infectious complications of bone marrow transplantation. *Oncology, 4* (2), 69-75.

ANTI-INFECTIVE THERAPY

Pamela J. Haylock, R.N., M.A.
Haylock - Cantril Associates, Woodside, CA

ANTI-INFECTIVE THERAPY

Pamela J. Haylock, R.N., M.A.
Haylock - Cantril Associates, Woodside, CA

INTRODUCTION

Neutropenia in the person with cancer is no longer an indication for hospitalization. In the event that fever develops, immediate medical assessment is indicated and will likely result in hospitalization and initiation of parenteral antibiotic therapy. After an infection is under control, parenteral antimicrobial therapy can be delivered in the home setting.

SCOPE OF THE PROBLEM

Infection is the major cause of morbidity and mortality among persons with cancer. Resistance to infection in people with cancer is altered by many interrelated factors including the cancer itself. Neutropenia related to cancer treatment modalities, drugs which modify the body's immune response (i.e., corticosteroids), and alterations in other nonspecific defenses such as skin integrity increase susceptibility to infection. Clinical presentation of infection may be altered in the neutropenic patient. Typical signs and symptoms are often absent. Progression from infection to sepsis can take place in a matter of hours. Mortality rates related to sepsis and septic shock range from 40% to 90%. The timeliness of recognition and appropriate intervention may determine the patient's fate.

CAUSES OF INFECTION IN THE IMMUNOCOMPROMISED PERSON WITH CANCER

Disease processes and side effects of treatment cause myelosuppression. The action of phagocytes is impaired in severe neutropenia secondary to chemotherapy, radiation therapy, or tumor invasion of the bone marrow. Neutrophil function may be altered in hematologic malignancies. Corticosteroids impair neutrophil migration and phagocytosis.

Lymphoid malignancies are related to abnormalities of cell-mediated immunity. The effects of chemotherapy make these individuals more susceptible to viral or fungal infections. Humoral immunity is also altered in people with hematologic malignancies and as a result, pyrogenic infections can occur even if the patient is not neutropenic.

PATHOGENS COMMON TO PERSONS WITH CANCER

The myelosuppressed patient is susceptible to infection from endogenous and exogenous microbial flora. When the integrity of the gastrointestinal tract is disrupted by local tumor invasion or the effects of cancer treatment and antibiotics, colonization and dissemination of pathogens can occur. Estimates indicate that more than 80% of infections in persons with cancer arise from endogenous microbial flora. Most of these infections are caused by *Psuedomonas aeruginosa, Escherichia coli, Klebsiella pneumonia,* and *Candida albicans.* (Pizzo and Young, 1985; Freifeld and Pizzo, 1991)

The most common bacterial pathogens in granulocytopenic persons are the gram-negative bacilli (*Pseudomonas, E-Coli,* and *Klebsiella pneumoniae*) and *Staphylococcus epidermidis.* Granulocytopenia and defects in phagocytic function of leukocytes increase susceptibility to certain fungi, protozoa and viruses, and infection caused by mycobacteria, *Listeria* and *Salmonella.* (Joshi, 1989)

Certain antineoplastic drugs, (daunorubicin, methotrexate and vincristine) inhibit phagocytosis and other granulocyte functions (Ehrke et al, 1989). Cyclophosphamide reduces antibody response and production. Cyclophosphamide suppresses delayed-type hypersensitivity reactions (Ehrke et al). Some antineoplastic agents inhibit granulocyte bactericidal activity. Dysfunction of cellular immunity is associated with certain malignant diseases, Hodgkin's Disease and Acquired Immune Deficiency Syndrome (AIDS), and other alterations in cellular immunity related to long-term immunosuppressive therapy i.e., organ transplant, acute lymphocytic leukemia in remission, and post-bone marrow transplantation.

Opportunistic pathogens which take advantage of defects in cellular immunity include bacteria (*Listeria monocytogenes,* nontyphosa Salmonella sp, Legionella sp, *M tuberculosis* and atypical mycobacteria and *Nocardia asteroides*); viruses (varicella zoster, cytomegalovirus, and herpes simplex); fungi (*C. neoformans, Histoplasma capsulatum,* and *Coccidioides immitis*); protozoa (*Pneumocystis carinii, Toxoplasma gondii,* and Cryptosporidium); and the helminth *Strongyloides stercoralis.* (Joshi, 1989)

Streptococcus pneumoniae and *Hemophilus influenzae* are encapsulated pathogens which frequently cause infections in persons with certain hematologic malignancies - multiple myeloma and chronic lymphocytic leukemia. Also at risk for infection with these organisms are individuals who have undergone splenectomy. Persons with chronic lymphocytic leukemia have a five-fold increased risk of infection due mainly to diminished circulating immune serum globulin. (Joshi, 1989)
Table 4.1 provides a summary of factors predisposing people with cancer to infection.

Special Pediatric Considerations
Children with acute lymphocytic leukemia who receive craniospinal irradiation have increased incidence of infections in the period following irradiation.

NURSING CONSIDERATIONS
Granulocytopenia is the single most important factor in determining the risk for infection and sepsis. The risk increases when the absolute granulocyte count falls below $500/mm^3$ and persists for more than 10 days. (Ellerhorst-Ryan, 1985) Nursing care planning for the patient who either

TABLE 4.1

Factors contributing to risk of infection

Factors	Examples
Humoral immunity defects	• Chronic lymphocytic leukemia, multiple myeloma
Cellular immunity defects	• Hodgkin's & non-Hodgkin's lymphoma, use of corticosteroids
Organ compromise due to obstruction	• Airway/bronchus obstruction in lung cancer, bowel obstruction in colo-rectal or metastatic sites
Granulocytopenia	• Acute leukemia, marrow suppression due to chemotherapy or radiation therapy
Disruption of integument &/or mucosal surfaces	• Mucositis & stomatitis from chemotherapy & radiation therapy
	• Desquamation from radiation, cutaneous metastases, invasive puncture/biopsy sites
Use of foreign devices	• Vascular access devices, urinary catheter
Central Nervous System	• Primary or metastatic brain tumor
Hypo-or asplenic (post-splenectomy) states	• Hodgkin's disease

Source: Oniboni, A.C. (1990). Infection in the Neutropenic Patient. Seminars in Oncology Nursing, 6(1), 50-60. Printed with permission.

is neutropenic or is likely to become neutropenic involves decreasing the risk of infection and/or increasing the likelihood of prompt recognition of signs of infection and initiation of treatment. (McNally and Stair, 1991) Laboratory values associated with immune response should be closely monitored. Optimal white blood cell levels are:

White blood cells (WBC) levels: 4000 to 10,000/uL

Differential WBC levels:

Neutrophils (polys, PMNs): 2500 to 6000/uL (40-60%)

Monocytes: 200 to 800/uL (4-8%)

Lymphocytes: 1800 to 4000/uL (20-40%)

There is a clear relationship between the level of circulating polymorphonuclear leukocytes (polys) (PMNs) and infection. The risk of infection rises when the absolute granulocyte count falls to or below 500/mm³ and increases with the duration of granulocytopenia. Granulocytes have a very short life span in circulation and their numbers can change drastically from day to day. Daily monitoring and calculation of the absolute granulocyte count is recommended during periods of anticipated leukopenia. The absolute granulocyte count is determined through calculations using both the total white blood cell count and the differential count which specifies the number of normal and abnormal or premature white blood cells by type.

Total WBC x percentage of granulocytes (polys/bands) = Absolute number of granulocytes for that day.

For example: Total WBC = 2500 cells/mm³
The differential is:

38% polys
12% bands
$\left. \right\}$ = 50% granulocytes

45% lymphocytes

1% eosinophils

1% basophils

3% monocytes

Polys and bands are granulocytes; 50% of the WBC's are granulocytes. To calculate the absolute number of granulocytes, multiply 50% or 0.50 times the total WBC of 2500.

2500 x 0.50 = 1250 = absolute granulocyte count for that day

ANTI-INFECTIVE THERAPY

The concept of anti-infective therapy must include aspects of prevention of infection. Essentially, all interventions fall within concepts of enhancing host defenses, minimizing alterations in natural barriers, and reducing the number of pathogenic organisms in the patient's environment. Despite major technological advances, fancy devices and sophisticated treatment strategies, the most important preventive intervention is simply vigorous handwashing by all care providers before and after each direct patient care activity. Other interventions include avoiding fresh flowers and cold water humidifiers in the "patient's" environment. Avoiding fresh salads and other raw foods (low pathogen diets) have not been scientifically documented as beneficial. Surveillance cultures of various body areas and fluids have been studied, but there is no consensus about their value in preventing infection.

Table 4.2 outlines measures to prevent or diminish chances of infection.

Table 4.2

Measures to Prevent or Diminish Chance of Infection

Intervention	Rationale

1. Daily "head to toe" assessment by patient and/or caregiver
  • Body temperature with oral thermometer
  • Systemic status: fever, chills, fatigue
  • Assess sites of peripheral and central vascular access devices
  • Assess biopsy sites, bone marrow biopsy/aspirate sites
	1. Monitor response to treatment and detect new area of infection, temperature elevation. In neutropenia, temperature elevation. In neutropenia, usual signs and symptoms of infection may be absent
	  • Avoid trauma to rectal area

2. Implement meticulous hygienic practices
  • Oral hygiene regimen (should be specific to clinical findings)
  Soft toothbrush and normal saline to clean teeth, gums and rinse every 2-4 hours while awake, and every 6 hours at night
  • Ongoing oral assessments
  • Perineal cleansing after defecation - ie.,
  Sitz bath or irrigate perineum with warm water
  • Daily bathing with special attention to intertiginous folds
  • Avoid douches and bubble baths
	2. Diminish surface pathogens and use this opportunity to inspect skin
	  • At least 40% of patients receiving chemotherapy have oral complications and oral cavity is very frequent site of infection and subsequent systemic infections-especially during therapy for acute leukemia

(continued)

Table 4.2

Measures to Prevent or Diminish Chance of Infection

Intervention	Rationale

3. Implement skin care regimen:
• Use mild soaps or plain water and rinse well-pat dry
• Use skin emollients after bathing
• If patient is undergoing or has had radiation therapy, some interventions will be specific to the treatment field:
    Avoid restrictive clothing
    Avoid irritants: soaps, deodorant, perfume, ointments, solvents, tape
    Assess daily for skin reactions, dry or wet desquamation
    Do not shave in the affected area
    Use plain water for cleansing
	3. Decrease drying, cracking amd other irritation to skin.

4. Implement measures to avoid accidental trauma to skin and mucous membrane: • Female patients should use sanitary napkins instead of tampon • Discontinue colostomy irrigation • Use extra caution when cutting toe- and fingernails • Wear shoes or slippers at all times	4. Diminish possible portals of entry for organisms.
5. Discuss sexuality and sexual practices: • Use adequate lubrication • Discuss contraceptives and infection risks	5. Minimize mucosal trauma during sexual activities: • Diaphragm increases the risk of cystitis • Progesterone increases risk for vaginal infections • May need to remove intrauterine device to decrease risk for endometrial infection
6. Promote pulmonary hygiene: • Encourage mobility • Encourage "cough and deep breathe" • Use incentive spirometer	6. Pneumonia can develop and without leukocytes, the only initial evidence may be rales.

(continued)

8. Promote high-calorie, high protein diet with vitamin C supplements.	8. Balanced nutrition promotes wound healing and restoration of cellular immunity. Protein and zinc deficiencies have negative effects on the cellular immune system.
9. Encourage low microbial neutropenic diet. Cooked foods only.	9. Normal intestinal flora may be altered and impair resistance to colonization with opportunistic organisms.
10. Avoid contact with communicable illnesses and persons who have recently been vaccinated with live or attenuated virus vaccines.	10. Minimize chances of communicable disease.

11. Remove all sources of stagnant water:
 	
    Denture cups
    Flower vases
    Water pitchers
    Humidifiers
    Soap dishes
	11. Stagnant water is a medium in which *Pseudomonas aeruginosa can* grow.

12. Encourage oral fluids to 3,000 cc/day unless contraindicated.	12. Avoid urinary stasis.

Source: Adapted from Volker (1992), Lazarus (1989), McNally & Stair (1991), and Brandt (1990).

COLONY STIMULATING FACTORS

The recent introduction of colony-stimulating factors (CSFs) has already influenced standard cytotoxic therapy. CSFs are a class of hormones that stimulate production of the cellular components of blood and accelerate leukocyte and granulocyte recovery. Since the risk of infection increases with the duration of neutropenia, the use of a CSF as an adjunct to chemotherapy can reduce neutropenia and diminish the risk of infection. By enhancing myeloid recovery, chemotherapy doses can be increased to much higher and more effective doses than are possible without CSFs. CSFs can reduce the incidence of fever with neutropenia and infections, and have been shown to decrease the total number of days of intravenous antibiotic therapy and hospitalization (Crawford et al, 1991). CSFs seem to have a positive influence on the quality of life in patients with chronic neutropenia (Fazio and Glaspy, 1991). Patients given CSF generally have fewer physician visits, fewer infectious episodes, and require fewer antibiotic regimens and hospitalizations during cancer treatment.

Granulocyte colony-stimulating factor (G-CSF) and granulocyte macrophage colony-stimulating factor (GM-CSF) have been introduced into clinical settings outside of clinical trials. Other colony-stimulating factors are likely to be available in the near future. CSF is started at a prescribed time after the completion of chemotherapy and continues for approximately two weeks. The actual duration of CSF therapy varies with protocol design. GM-CSF and G-CSF can be self-administered subcutaneously or can be given intravenously. Side effects are dose-related: higher doses elicit more severe side effects. Side effects of GM-CSF are generally mild and include low-grade fever, mild chills, headache, myalgias, bone pain, nausea, reduced appetite, skin rash, thrombocytopenia and fatigue (Haeuber, 1989; Vadhan-Raj, 1989). At high doses (>32 micrograms/kg/day) fluid retention, pleuropericarditis and thrombosis of central venous catheters have been reported (Vadhan-Raj). Side effects of G-CSF are less remarkable and mainly involve bone pain and myalgias with low grade fever (Haeuber; Vadhan-Raj). Other side effects including skin rash, flare-up of psoriasis, vasculitis, and splenomegaly have been anecdotally reported (Vadhan-Raj). Maximum tolerated doses of GM-CSF range from 16-32 micrograms/kg/day (Glaspy and Golde, 1989). A maximal tolerated dose for G-CSF has not been identified (Freifeld and Pizzo, 1991) though trials have included infusions of 1-60 micrograms/kg/day (Gabrilove et al, 1988).

CSFs may be administered safely in the home setting. Patient and family education provided by the nurse includes (ONS, 1989; Melone et al, 1991):

- Review the specific agents making up the planned treatment regimen, the treatment schedule and the method of administration;
- Use of audiovisual aids and printed materials to reinforce content;

- Preparation steps;
  - premedication to reduce or minimize hypersensitivity reactions
  - handwashing before and after
  - gentle vial rotation to dissolve powder
  - avoiding interchanging manufacturer brand with same patient
  - aseptic intramuscular or subcutaneous injection techniques
  - rotation of injection sites (alternating sites on anterior thigh and abdomen for subcutaneous injections);
  - proper storage techniques-refrigeration and avoid freezing or room temperature storage;
- Assessment of injection sites;
- Disposal of needles and syringes;
- Management of accidental spillage of the drug;
- Avoidance of steroids, nonsteroidal anti-inflammatory agents;
- Avoidance of medications containing aspirin which might alter the immune response;
- Avoidance of topical ointments;
- Scheduling administration times to minimize interference with daily activities, secondary fatigue and other side effects;
- Review of anticipated side effects and symptom management;
- Review of when and who to contact for questions and concerns;
- Supply printed educational material to reinforce instructions

OTHER MEASURES FOR INFECTION PROPHYLAXIS

Immunoprophylaxis involves manipulation of the immune system to enable it to resist infection more efficiently. Intravenous gamma globulin increases the total IgG level which reduces the incidence of infection when hypogammaglobulinemia is a component of the underlying pathophysiology. Chronic lymphocytic or myelogenous leukemia, multiple myeloma, and some lymphomas are known to involve hypogammaglobulinemia. Other agents which affect immune function include lithium carbonate and some vaccines. Lithium carbonate seems to accelerate hematopoietic recovery after cytotoxic chemotherapy. Use of vaccines for pneumococcus, meningococcus, and Haemophilus influenzae B are thought to prevent these infections in persons who have undergone splenectomy.

Antibacterial prophylaxis with oral nonabsorbable antibiotics (vancomycin, gentamicin, polymyxin, nystatin) reduces endogenous gastrointestinal flora. These antibiotics are generally unpalatable and cause unpleasant side effects including nausea, vomiting and diarrhea, making patient compliance problematic. The expense of these drugs combined with questionable compliance limits the usefulness of these regimens.

Gastrointestinal decontamination using trimethoprim-sulfamethoxazole is being studied. This regimen preserves anaerobic flora but reduces the aerobic bacterial population.

Antiviral and antifungal prophylaxis have been suggested but effectiveness is not documented. When susceptible fungi are eradicated, an overgrowth of more resistant fungi is likely to occur. Oral and parenteral acyclovir has been used to prevent herpetic infections in patients during induction chemotherapy and bone marrow transplantation. Acyclovir resistance has been observed, especially in patients who have received several treatment courses. None of the available antiviral agents or interferons are effective in preventing infection with cytomegalovirus (CMV) (Pizzo and Young, 1985).

FEVER IN THE PERSON WITH CANCER

Fever can occur as a result of tumor-associated factors, reactions to blood component transfusions, and reactions to drugs – particularly amphotericin and some types of biologic response modifiers (e.g., colony stimulating factors, interleukins). Nevertheless, fever in a neutropenic patient must be considered indicative of infection until proven otherwise. Suspicion of infection in the person with cancer requires urgent assessment and intervention. Fever in the neutropenic cancer patient represents an absolute emergency (Lazarus, et al, 1989).

Clinical Evaluation

The usual signs and symptoms of infection may be masked. Without granulocytes, purulence or fluctuance and other cardinal symptoms may not develop. When fever develops without an apparent etiology (drug therapy, tumor, transfusions), all portals of pathogen entry must be examined. The initial clinical evaluation must include skin with particular attention to fingerstick or venipuncture sites, biopsy sites, and skin folds, i.e., breasts, axilla and groin. The perirectal area should be assessed: a history of hemorrhoids places neutropenic patients, especially those with leukemia, at particular risk for infection. Oral cavity examination should include the teeth and gingivae, tongue and floor of the mouth, nasopharynx and sinuses. Abdominal distension or tenderness may signify an acute surgical abdomen caused by the underlying cancer or cancer treatment. A person with cancer can have a more common abdominal problem like appendicitis and cholecystitis. Table 4.3 outlines the clinical evaluation of the febrile patient. Table 4.4 identifies the organisms responsible for the majority of infections in cancer patients.

Initiation of Treatment-Antibiotic Therapy

Antibiotic therapy should be initiated (after appropriate cultures have been obtained) promptly in febrile neutropenic patients. There is general consensus that antibiotic therapy should be started before microbial culture results are available. Empiric (meaning before an infectious agent is identified) use of broad-spectrum antibacterial agents represents a major

TABLE 4.3

Clinical Evaluation of the Febrile Neutropenic Patient

Assessment	Assess for
Skin	• Erythema, pain and/or pus at venipuncture sites
	• Erythema, pain and/or pus at sites of other invasive procedures
	• Skin eruptions, erythema at skin fold and/or intertiginous areas
	• Dry and/or wet desquamation secondary to radiation
Vascular Access Devices	• Blood for culture from each lumen and the peripheral vein
	• Fluid expressed from catheter exit site for culture
Eyes	• Ophthalmology consult for fundoscopic exam, dilation and indirect opthalmascopic exam to detect fungal infection
Oral Cavity	• Mouth, tongue, teeth, oropharynx
CNS	• Neurologic exam
Perirectal area	• Perianal lesions - especially common with history of hemorrhoids. Gentle inspection and palpation, questions related to pain on defecation, mucosal tear
Lungs	• Rales, cough, or sputum
Abdomen	• Distension and tenderness
Other sites	
Esophagus	• Endoscopic exam for esophageal lesions
Urinary tract	• Frequency and/or dysuria
Stool	• Diarrhea-culture for bacteria, virus, parasites
Pleural fluid (if available)	• Culture
Peritoneal fluid (if available)	• Culture
Ommaya Reservoir	• Potential entry for skin pathogens

TABLE 4.4

Organisms Responsible for Majority of Infections in Cancer Patients

Bacteria	Fungi	Viruses
Gram-negative	Aspergillus sp.	Herpes Simplex
Klebsiella	Candida sp.	Cytomegalovirus
Enterobacter	Torulopsis glabrata	Hepatitis A,B, and non-A, non-B
Serratia	Zygomycoses	Varicella Zoster
E Coli	Cryptococcus neoformans	
Pseudomonas aeruginosa		
Proteus		
Gram-positive		
Staphyloccus aureas		
Staphylococcus-epidermidis		
Streptococcus		
Corynebacteria		
Clostridia difficile		
Enterococcus		
Other		
Mycobacteria sp.		
Legionella sp.		

Adapted from Lazarus (1989), Gucalp (1991) and Volker (1992).

advance in the management of infection in persons with cancer. Without immediate antibiotic therapy, a mortality rate within 48 hours of 70% of febrile neutropenic patients has been documented (Bodey et al, 1985). There is no consensus about which antibiotic to use or whether single versus combinations of antibiotics should be used in empiric therapy.

The goal of empiric antibiotic therapy is to protect the patient from complications of untreated bacterial infection. Historically, the predominant organisms responsible for infections in the neutropenic population were gram-negative bacteria – *Escherichia coli, Klebsiella pneumoniae,* and *Pseudomonas aeruginosa* (Gucalp, 1991). In recent years, gram-positive organisms have been the major pathogens responsible for infection in this population. Empiric antibiotic therapy has generally combined an aminoglycoside and an extended spectrum penicillin (carbenicillin, ticarcillin, or piperacillin) which provided coverage against a wide array of potential pathogens. During the past decade, new antimicrobials have been developed which offer alternatives to aminoglycoside-containing regimens and can be used as single agents (monotherapy) in empirical management of the febrile neutropenic patient. Other agents are available in an oral preparation and may facilitate outpatient management of cancer patients (Frefield and Pizzo, 1991).

There are four categories of antibiotic regimens suggested for empiric antibiotic therapy in the febrile neutropenic patient (Armstrong, Bodey, et al, 1990).

1. Aminoglycoside plus anti-pseudomonal beta-lactam.

Anti-pseudomonal penicillins or third generation cephalosporins are beta-lactam antibiotics. The aminoglycoside seems to prevent development of resistance to the beta-lactams. These combinations work synergistically against gram-negative bacilli. The major disadvantages include nephrotoxicity and ototoxicity. The efficacy of this combination is dose-dependent: suboptimal dosing limits the efficacy of the regimen.

2. Combination of two beta-lactams.

Combinations of third-generation cephalosporins (i.e., ceftazidime or cefoperazone) and antipseudomonal penicillins (i.e., ticarcillin or pipercillin) are as effective as aminoglycoside-containing regimens but have less toxicity. Limitations of these combinations include:

- Expense of the drugs;
- The use of one type of antibiotic may increase the emergence of resistant organisms;
- Some beta-lactams cause or prolong neutropenia;
- The double beta-lactam regimen increases the risk of developing fungal infections.

Even with these limitations, double beta-lactam regimens provide an option for patients who have compromised renal status, the elderly, and patients who are receiving other nephrotoxic drugs such as cisplatin, cyclosporins, amphotericin B, or those who have impaired eighth-nerve function.

3. Vancomycin plus Aminoglycoside and Antipseudomonal beta-lactam.

With the increased use of indwelling vascular access catheters came the increased incidence of gram-positive infections. These catheters provide a portal of entry for skin flora such as Staphylococcus. Empiric antibiotic regimens designed to cover gram-negative organisms are not effective against all gram-positive pathogens. These organisms are often sensitive only to vancomycin (Gulcap, 1991). Vancomycin is expensive and there is concern about its empiric use. It has been documented that there is no difference in the morbidity rate in patients who received vancomycin empirically and those in whom vancomycin was started after positive cultures were obtained (Lazarus, et al, 1989). However, if methicillin-resistant *S. epidermidis* or *S. aureus* is suspected-i.e., is known to be a pathogen within the patient's health care facility, vancomycin is the drug of choice for empiric therapy. Vancomycin can be discontinued should culture results fail to show gram-positive cocci (Lazarus et al).

4. Monotherapy.

Monotherapy - use of a single drug - had high failure rates, and resistance to beta-lactam antibiotics emerged during early trials. New beta-lactam antibiotics (cefoperazone, cefazidime) and carbapenems (imipenem) have spectrums which include the common gram-negative pathogens and are being tested in new clinical trials. Results, so far, still seem to favor combination therapy (Gulcap, 1991). Imipenem is not effective against non-aeruginosa pseudomonads, or methicillin-resistant S. aureus. Many coagulase-negative staphylococci and P. aeruginosa frequently develop resistance to it (Freifeld and Pizzo, 1991).

Regardless of the regimen implemented, bacteriostatic antibiotics (tetracyclines, erythromycin, chloramphenicol, etc.) should be avoided. They are not beneficial in the absence of granulocytes and when given concomitantly, reduce the efficacy of the bactericidal antibiotic (Grunwald, 1991).

After Initial Management

After a specific pathogen is isolated, antibiotic therapy can be modified to provide optimal response to therapy with minimal toxicity. Broad-spectrum coverage must be maintained to prevent secondary bacterial infections.

Antibacterial therapy is usually discontinued after 5 to 7 days if the patient has an adequate granulocyte count (in excess of 500 micrograms/ L) and remains afebrile and free of infection (Lazarus et al, 1989). There is no consensus about appropriate management in instances of persistent granulocytopenia when the patient is afebrile. There are advocates of continuing therapy (Lazarus et al) while others favor stopping antibiotics when the patient is stable (Gucalp, 1991). Patients in whom positive cultures were obtained are likely to be treated for a total of 10 to 14 days, or until the granulocyte count exceeds 500 micrograms/L, whichever is longer (Lazarus et al).

Persistent or New Fever - Fungal Infections

Continued granulocytopenia is usually associated with the emergence of non-bacterial opportunistic infections. Successful antibiotic management of bacterial infections has been followed by the appearance of fungal infections – particularly *Candida* and *Aspergillus*. Fungal infections are a major cause of morbidity and mortality in people with cancer. Since methods of diagnosing early fungal infections are not generally available, it is recommended that persistently febrile (in excess of 5 to 7 days) neutropenic patients continue on antibiotic therapy with the addition of the antifungal agent amphotericin B (Gucalp 1991; Lazarus, et al, 1989). If institution of antifungal therapy is delayed until positive blood culture or skin biopsy culture, the patient is more likely to develop disseminated infection before adequate tissue levels of amphotericin B can be achieved (Lazarus et al). There are reports of fungal organisms developing resistance to amphotericin B. Alternative antifungal agents include 5-fluorocytosine, miconazole, fluconazole and itraconazole. These agents, with the exception of fluconazole, are administered intravenously. Fluconazole is available in both oral and parenteral preparations.

Rigors are a well-known complication of amphotericin B. Intravenous meperidine or dantrolene may diminish or prevent rigors. Other toxicities related to amphotericin B include renal dysfunction, fever, thrombocytopenia, and pulmonary infiltrates. A test dose of amphotericin is recommended. Amphotericin B can be prepared with 40 to 50 mg (0.6 mg/kg) in 100 to 250 ml of 5% dextrose/water. A test dose containing 10 mg amphotericin B is infused over 2 hours. If this test dose is tolerated, the remainder of the drug can be given. Other test dose regimens use a 1 mg test dose with gradual incremental increases in daily doses to 0.5 mg/kg/d. If there is a clinical response - the patient becomes afebrile - amphotericin B is continued until a cumulative dose ranging from 500 mg to 3 g is reached (Lazarus, 1989).

Viral Infections

Herpes viruses are the most common viral pathogens in persons with cancer. Herpes simplex virus (HSV) types 1 and 2, varicella-zoster virus (VZV), and cytomegalovirus (CMV) cause the most morbidity. Acyclovir limits the clinical severity of many infections due to HSV and VZV, but acyclovir and other available antiviral agents cannot eliminate latent viral infections. Acyclovir has little activity against existing CMV. Acyclovir given prophylactically to bone marrow transplant patients has decreased the occurrence of VZV and CMV disease during the post-transplant period (Freifeld and Pizzo, 1991).

Ganciclovir is effective against HSV types 1 and 2, VZV, and possibly CMV. Neutropenia is a common, dose-limiting toxicity of ganciclovir (Freifeld and Pizzo, 1991).

Foscarnet is useful in the treatment of acyclovir-resistant HSV. There have been some clinical responses to foscarnet in transplant recipients and CMV infections. Its efficacy in the treatment of CMV retinitis in AIDS patients has been demonstrated. (Freifeld and Pizzo, 1991).

Granulocyte transfusions

Granulocyte transfusions are associated with significant complications, including transmission of infection, development of pulmonary infiltrates, and accelerated alloimmunization. For these reasons, granulocyte transfusions are generally reserved for situations in which the patient is anticipated to have prolonged neutropenia and has persistent gram-negative bacteremia (Lazarus: Erickson, 1990).

Polypharmacy

Most people with cancer are treated with a wide variety of drugs. In addition to antineoplastic drugs, there is a good chance that the person with cancer is also taking prescribed medication for non-cancer reasons – i.e., anti-hypertensives, sedatives, allopurinol, antidepressants, antibiotics and over-the-counter medications containing aspirin and other salicylates, analgesics, acetaminophen and non-steroidal anti-inflammatory agents. Drug interactions, pharmacodynamics and pharmacokinetics of each drug must be considered.

The fact that the majority of people with cancer are over 50 is a significant factor in drug selection and overall treatment plans. After the age of 60, some basic changes occur in physiologic functions. Glomerular filtration rate, cardiac index, and breathing capacity all decline. The percentage of body water decreases as does lean body mass. Hepatic blood flow diminishes to half what is was at ages 20-30.

Additive, overlappping, and/or interactive toxicities of all medications the patient is currently taking, or has taken previously, must be considered in the development of the treatment plan and also assessment parameters. Additive/overlapping toxicity is a toxicity which is common to both drugs

TABLE 4.5

Drugs which cause renal impairment

Antimicrobials	Antineoplastics
Trimethoprim	Corticosteroids
Cefoxitin	Mitomycin C
Flucytosine	Cisplatin
Rifampin	Streptozocin
Ampicillin	Interferon
Aminoglycosides	Cyclosporine
Amphotericin B	Semustine
Beta Lactams	Methotrexate (high dose)
Erythromycin	Interleukin-2
Acyclovir	

Source: Finley, R.S. (1990). The patient's other medicines: A pharmacology overview-Antimicrobial therapy in patients receiving cancer chemotherapy. Oncology Nursing Society Congress. Reprinted with Permission.

that may worsen following concomitant therapy. Interactive toxicity is a toxicity produced by one drug which may increase the chance or severity of toxicity produced by a second drug.

Certain antineoplastic and antimicrobials cause renal impairment. Risk factors for renal dysfunction in connection with drug therapy include age, concomitant nephrotoxic drugs, prior renal impairment, dehydration, and cell lysis. Many of these agents are excreted via the kidneys. Table 4.5 identifies the drugs which are known to cause renal impairment.

Decreased renal function may lead to increases in serum and tissue concentrations of drugs which are normally excreted primarily via the kidneys resulting in other dose-related toxicities. Antimicrobials secreted via the kidneys include acyclovir, the aminoglycosides, B-lactams, vancomycin, flucytosine, and ganciclovir. Antineoplastics excreted through the kidneys include bleomycin, carboplatin, cisplatin, etoposide, mithramycin, and methotrexate (Bartlett, 1991).

Manifestations of renal dysfunction include increased serum creatinine and BUN, decreased urinary output, proteinuria, decrease in measured creatinine clearance, and electrolyte imbalance. In general, renal dysfunction can be managed and is reversible. Precautions include hydration and adjustment of doses depending on the drugs selected. In some instances, dialysis is implemented as a supportive measure (Finley, 1990).

Antimicrobials and antineoplastics are capable of inducing liver damage. Risk factors associated with hepatic dysfunction include prior dysfunction and concomitant hepatotoxins. Hepatic dysfunction can significantly decrease the metabolism of agents which are primarily metabolized by the liver allowing the drug to remain active, again, resulting in additional toxicities.

Table 4.6 lists the drugs which cause liver complications in persons with cancer.

TABLE 4.6

Drugs Which Cause Hepatic Dysfunction

Antimicrobials	Antineoplastics
Beta Lactams	Asparaginase
Erythromycin	Carmustine
Tetracycline	Cyclosporine
Sulfas	Chlorambucil
Isoniazid	Cisplatin
Rifampin	Dacarbazine
Ketoconazole	Daunorubicin
Flucytosine	Doxorubicin
	Methotrexate
	Mercaptopurine
	Mithramycin
	Thioguanine
	Vinblastine

Drugs Metabolized Primarily by the Liver

Antimicrobials	Antineoplastics
Chloramphenicol	Busulfan
Ketoconazole	Chlorambucil
Rifampin	Cyclophosphamide
Isoniazid	Cytarabine
Metronidazole	Dacarbazine
Ketoconazole	Fluorouracil
Interferons	
Mitomycin	
Carmustine	
Mercaptopurine	
Thioguanine	
Streptozocin	
Thiotepa	

Finley, R.S. (1990) The patient's other medicines: A pharmacology overview-Antimicrobial therapy in patients receiving cancer chemotherapy. Oncology Nursing Society Congress. Reprinted with permission.

TABLE 4.7

Drug Interactions and Clinical Significance

Interacting Drugs	Effects	Assessment / Monitoring
Aminoglycosides/ cisplatin	Increased nephrotoxicity	Serum creatinine, BUN,creatinine clearance; monitor serum aminoglycoside levels; hydration and diuresis pre- and post- cisplatin
	Increased ototoxicity	Clinical assessment of hearing; serial audiograms; monitor serum aminoglycoside levels
Amphotericin B/ cisplatin	Increased nephrotoxicity	monitor serum creatinine, BUN, cisplatin creatinine clearance, hydration/diureses
	Increased electrolyte imbalance (Hypokalemia and hypomagnesemia)	monitor serum potassium, magnesium, phosphate, replace electrolytes
Ketoconazole/ cyclosporin	Increased cyclosporine levels leading to increased nephrotoxicity	monitor cyclosporine levels, serum creatinine, BUN, creatinine clearance
Erythromycin/ cyclosporin	Increased cyclosporine levels leading to increased nephrotoxicity	monitor cyclosporine levels, serum creatinine, BUN, creatinine clearance

Finley, R.S. (1990). The patient's other medicines: A pharmacology overview-Antimicrobial therapy in patients receiving cancer chemotherapy. Oncology Nursing Society Congress. Reprinted with permission.

Even though many antimicrobials are metabolized by the liver or excreted via the biliary tract, few require dose modifications even with known hepatic dysfunction. Doses are usually modified only if there is concurrent renal dysfunction and/or the liver disease is acute or associated with severe hepatic failure manifested as ascites or jaundice (Bartlett, 1991).

While liver and kidney function are most crucial, other polypharmacy issues include drugs which cause bone marrow suppression and other hematologic effects, gastrointestinal intolerance, febrile reactions, neurotoxicity, and dermatologic and allergic reactions. Appropriate premedication assessments will establish baseline information. Modifications in drug choice, dose, and administration schedules may be indicated.

For the individual with cancer, the most significant potential drug interactions involve antimicrobials and antineoplastics. In the febrile or infected neutropenic patient, these considerations take on added importance. The most clinically significant drug interactions in this patient population are outlined in Table 4.7.

HOME ANTIMICROBIAL THERAPY

Initial parenteral antimicrobial therapy for the febrile, neutropenic patient should be managed in a hospital setting. Home parenteral antimicrobial therapy is preferred for managing a course of therapy for infections which require prolonged, repeated, or short-term antibiotic or other antimicrobial agents. Criteria for patient selection for home parenteral antimicrobial therapy include (Dolbee and Creason, 1988):

1. Signs and symptoms of infection are under control.

2. Other aspects of the patient's care plan can be monitored and /or performed in the home.

3. The patient and family understand and agree with the plan for home therapy.

4. The patient and/or caregiver can perform necessary procedures for home therapy.

5. The patient has peripheral veins suited for repeated cannulizations or has a vascular access device in place.

6. The patient has suitable home environment for therapy (i.e., refrigerator, freezer, telephone, and transportation).

7. The arrangement of payment for supplies, medication, skilled nursing visits, laboratory tests, and clinic appointments is agreeable to the patient and family.

The frequency of nursing visits will vary in frequency from three times a day to once a week to once a month, depending on the phase of treatment (acute vs. chronic), the type of vascular access in place (peripheral, central, or PICC) and related dressing requirements, the patient's clinical findings, and frequency of laboratory monitoring required in each situation (McNally & Stair, 1990).

During each visit, the nurse monitors vital signs, laboratory test results, equipment operation, supplies, drug effects and signs and symptoms of complications.

The nurse is responsible for ensuring that medications and supplies are stored and mixed according to pharmaceutical guidelines.

The simplest, least costly, drug delivery system is gravity infusion which is easily adapted to the home. However, with antibiotics in which flow rate is a critical factor or those that could cause phlebitis, an infusion, controller or pump is preferred. Variables related to drug selection for home infusion plans should include dosing intervals and potential adverse effects. A drug that requires only once or twice daily administration is ideal in the home setting.

Recommended refrigeration temperature of 36-44° F can be achieved in most home refrigerators. Some antibiotics are stable for 30 days and are available in prepared frozen piggyback solutions. Proper thawing techniques must be used to prevent inactivation or degradation. Generally, the antibiotic should be left at room temperature until it is completely thawed.

With most antibiotics, small parenteral bags can be thawed in advance and refrigerated for use the next day (Kasmer, Hoisington and Yukniewics, 1987).

Patient and family education is critical to the safe administration of antibiotics in the home setting. The individual responsible for the administration procedure and monitoring – either patient, caregiver or both, must be assessed for psychomotor skill, dexterity, vision, basic mathematical skills, reading ability, and ability to understand and follow instructions. Many homecare agencies have implemented patient-provider contracts as a means of enhancing patient compliance to therapy. A teaching care plan and patient/caregiver demonstration of appropriate skills is necessary for successful home management (Coker & Lampert, 1990). Teaching plans must include:

- vascular access device and site care

- signs and symptoms of infection and recurrent infection: self-monitoring

- drug admixture procedures

- drug administration techniques

- appropriate drug storage

- potential complications – recognition and intervention

- infusion device operation if applicable

- troubleshooting and problem solving

- when and who to contact with questions and concerns

- written instructions

Quality assurance plans should incorporate identified outcome criteria in six areas of home IV antibiotic care (Dolbee & Creason, 1988):

1. Infusion-related complications

2. Drug-related complications

3. Home care management

4. Psychosocial response of patient/caregiver

5. Cost

6. Recovery

SUMMARY

Individuals with cancer are at considerable risk for the development of infections. Appropriate nursing interventions, whether in the in-patient, ambulatory, or homecare setting must incorporate sound patient/family education strategies. Self-care instructions are targeted toward prevention of infection. Self-monitoring is directed at recognizing early signs and symptoms of infection. The patient and/or caregiver are most likely to notice early signs and symptoms of infection. Failure to treat infection early can result in fatal complications. On the other hand, prompt recognition and timely, effective intervention can have a very positive impact on the quality and quantity of life for the patient. The nurse must prepare the patient and family for the responsibilities expected in the homecare setting.

REFERENCES

Antman, K.S., Griffin, J.D., Elias, A., Socinski, M.A., Ryan, L., Cannistra, S.A., Oette, D., Whitley, M., Frei, E., Schnipper, L.E. (1988) Effect of recombinant human granulocyte-macrophage colony-stimulating factor on chemotherapy-induced myelosupression. *New Engl Journal Med, 319* (10), 593-598.

Bartlett, J.G. (1991) *Pocketbook of Infectious Disease Therapy.* Baltimore: Williams & Wilkins.

Bodey, G.P., Jadeja, L., and Elting, L (1985) Pseudomonas bacteremia: Retrospective analysis of 410 episodes. *Arch Inter Med, 145*:1621-1629.

Brandt, B. (1990) Nursing protocol for the patient with neutropenia. *Oncology Nursing Forum, Supplement 17* (1), 9-15.

Coker, M., and Lampert, A. (1990) Teaching checklist for home infusion therapy. *Oncology Nursing Forum, 17*(6) 923-926.

Crawford, J. Ozer, H., Stoller, R., Johnson, D., Lyman, G., Tabbarra, I., Kris, M., Grous, J., Picozzi, V., Rausch, G., Smith, R., Gradishar, W., Yahanda, A., Vincent, M., Stewart, M., and Glaspy, J. (1991) Reduction by granulocyte colony-stimulating factor of fever and neutropenia induced by chemotherapy in patients with small-cell lung cancer. *New Engl Journal Med, 325*(3), 164-170.

David J. (1992) Organs and cells of the immune system. (In) Rubenstein, E. and Federman, D.D., (Eds). *Medicine,* New York: Scientific American, Inc. Section 6, Immunology.

Dolbee, S.F. and Creason, N.S. (1988) Outcome criteria for the patient using antibiotic therapy at home. *Home Health-Care Nurse, 6*(4), 22-29.

Ehrke, M.J., Mihich, E., Berd, D., D., and Mastrangelo, M.J. (1989) Effects of anticancer drugs on the immune system in humans. *Seminars in Oncology, 16*(3), 230-253.

Ellerhorst-Ryan, J.M. (1985) Complications of the myeloproliferative system: infection and sepsis. *Seminars in Oncology Nursing, 1*(4), 244-250.

Erickson, J.M. (1990) Blood support for the myelosuppressed patient. *Seminars in Oncology Nursing, 6*(1),61-66.

Fazio, M.T. and Glaspy, J.A. (1991) The impact of granulocyte colony-stimulating factor on quality of life in patients with severe chronic neutropenia. *Oncology Nursing Forum, 18*(8), 1411-1414.

Finley, R.S. (1990) The patient's other medicines: A pharmacology overview-antimicrobial therapy in patients receiving cancer chemotherapy. Presented during Pre-Congress Session, Oncology Nursing Society Congress, May 15.

Freifeld, A. and Pizzo, P. (1991) New developments in the antimicrobial supportive care of the immunocompromised patient. *PPO Updates, 5*(10).

Gabrilove, J.L., Jakubowski, A., Scher, H., Sternberg, C., Wong, G., Grous, J., Yagoda, A., Fain, K., Moore, M.A.S., Clarkson, F., Oettgen, H.F., Alton, K., Welte, K., Souza, L. (1988) Effect of granulocyte colony-stimulating factor on neutropenia and associated morbidity due to chemotherapy for transitional-cell carcinoma of the urothelium. *New Engl Journal Med, 318*(22), 1414-22.

Gallucci, B. (1987). The immune system and cancer. *Onc Nurs Forum,* 14(6), Supple, 3-12.

Glapsy, J.A. and Golde, D.W. (1989) Clinical applications of the myeloid growth factors. *Seminars in Hematology, 26*(2), Suppl 2 (April):14-17.

Grunwald, H.W. (1991) Management of the febrile neutropenic patient with cancer: The article reviewied. *Oncology, 5*(7), 148.

Gulcap, R. (1991) Management of the febrile neutropenic patient with cancer. *Oncology, 5*(7), 137-144.

Haeuber D. (1989) Recent advances in the management of biotherapy-related side effects: Flu-like syndrome. *The Biotherapy of Cancer III,* Symposium Proceedings, May 19, San Francisco.

Joshi, J.H. (1989) Epidemiology of infections in cancer patients. *Mediguide to Infectious Diseases. 9*(2), 1-5.

Kasmer, R.J., Hoisington, L.M., Yukniewicz. (1987) Home parenteral antibiotic therapy. II. Drug preparation and administration consider-ations. *Home Healthcare Nurse, 5*(1), 19-29.

Lazarus, H.M., Creger, R.J., and Gerson, S.L. (1989) Infectious emergen-cies in oncology patients. *Seminars in Oncology, 16*(6), 543-560.

McNally, J.C. and Stair, J. (1991) Potential for infection. (In) McNally JC, Somerville ET, Miaskowski C, Rostad M. (eds) *Guidelines for Oncology Nursing Practice* (2nd Ed), Philadelphia: W.B. Saunders.

McNally, J.C. and Stair, J. (1990) "Home care" pp. 1106-1131. (In) Groenwald, S.L., Frogge, M.H., Goodman, M., and Yarbro, C.H., (eds.) *Cancer Nursing: Principles and Practice,* (2nd Ed.) Boston: Jones and Bartlett.

Melone, L., Anderson-Drevs, K., Jassak, P., Quirch, C., Melone, L. (1991) A teaching booklet for patients receiving GM-CSF therapy. *Oncology Nursing Forum,* 18(3), 593-597.

Nossal, G.J.V. (1987) Current concepts: Immunology. The basic components of the immune system. *New Engl Journal Med, 316*(21), 1320-1325.

Oncology Nursing Society. (1989) *Biological Response Modifier Guidelines:* Recommendations for Nursing Education and Practice. Pittsburgh: Oncology Nursing Society.

Oniboni, A.C. (1990) Infection in the neutropenic patient. *Seminars in Oncology Nursing, 6*(1), 50-60.

Pizzo, P.A., and Young, R. (1985) Infections in the cancer patient. (In) DeVita, V.T., Hellman, S., Rosenberg, S.A. (Eds) *Cancer Principles and Practice of Oncology* (2nd ed). Vol. 2. Philadelphia: J.B. Lippincott. Ch. 52, 1963-1998.

Rostad, M.E. (1990) Management of myelosuppression in the patient with cancer. *Oncology Nursing Forum, 17*(1) Supple, 4-8.

Vadhan-Raj, S. (1989) Biotherapy with colony stimulating factors. *The Biotherapy of Cancer III.* Symposium Proceedings, May 19, 1989, San Francisco.

Volker, D.L. (1992) Infection in the cancer patient with an ostomy. *Journal of ET Nursing, 19*(1), 17-23.

Weeks, JC, Tierney MR, Weinstein MC (1991). Cost effectiveness of prophylactic intravenous immune globulin in chronic lymphocytic leukemia. *N Engl J Med, 325*: 81-86.

NUTRITIONAL MANAGEMENT OF THE CANCER PATIENT

Julie Hulsey Alles, R.D., L.D., C.N.S.D.
NMC Homecare, McKinney, Texas

NUTRITIONAL MANAGEMENT OF THE CANCER PATIENT

Julie Hulsey Alles, R.D., L.D., C.N.S.D.

NMC Homecare, McKinney, Texas

INTRODUCTION

The importance of the relationship between nutrition and cancer has been recognized for many years. Cancers exert negative effects on nutritional status. This may be due to the type and location of the cancer as well as the oncologic therapy employed. Surgery, radiation therapy and chemotherapy predictably increase nutrient requirements and, at the same time, interfere with the patient's ability to eat. Malnutrition may result from intense efforts to eradicate the malignancy by combinations of antineoplastic modalities. Consequently, potential benefits of oncologic therapy can be lost because of induced malnutrition (Copeland & Souba, 1988).

Cancer cachexia describes a group of symptoms and signs - anorexia, weakness, tissue wasting, and organ dysfunction. Cachexia, common in patients with advanced metastatic disease, occurs in patients with localized disease. The relationship of cachexia to tumor burden, disease stage, and cell type is inconsistent. No single theory satisfactorily explains the cachectic state. (Daley, et. al. 1990) It is likely to be a complex interaction of factors. These include: mechanical obstruction of the gastrointestinal tract, test abnormalities, malabsorption, and alterations in energy expenditure associated with malignancy. In addition, glucose recycling and futile cycles resulting from the predominant anaerobic metabolism of glucose by the tumor, as well as excessive lipid mobilization resulting from an increase in lipolytic activity of the serum may occur. Dissolution of host lean body mass continues unabated in the cancer patient and is the most obvious clinical manifestation of cancer cachexia.

Nutritional therapy is an important supportive measure for the patient undergoing antineoplastic treatment. It increases the well-being of the patient and may permit the administration of more intensive therapies. There is no conclusive evidence that adequate nutritional support preferentially feeds the tumor and results in increased tumor growth in humans. However, there is good evidence that effective nutritional repletion can reduce postoperative complications and mortality rates after surgery in severely malnourished patients. (Daley, et. al. 1990) It has been proposed that aggressiveness of feeding should be dictated by the type of antineoplastic therapy that the patient is receiving. (DeWys, 1985) Aggressive feeding may accompany curative or ablative chemotherapy but a more moderate nutritional regimen would be in order for palliative care. (Wachsman & Hardin, 1988)

The importance of an adequate nutritional status exists due to the recognition that nutrition is an integral part of healing, resisting infections, and maintaining a sense of well-being. The goals of nutrition support in the cancer patient are to achieve and maintain desirable weight and to prevent or correct nutritional imbalances and deficiencies.

In addition, a feeling of "well-being" contributes to maximum physical, social and psychologic function (Paloc, 1985).

The purposes of nutritional assessment are: to recognize early and subtle malnutrition, to correct the problem, to assist the patient through the metabolic insult of treatment, to reduce morbidity and mortality and to minimize loss of patient strength. However, nutritional assessment is complex due to difficulty in determining whether the altered nutritional assessment parameters are related to nutrient deprivation or the effect of the disease (Douglass, 1984).

Pediatric Nutrition Support

Specialists in child health have long recognized the contribution that proper nutrition makes to normal growth and development. Attention has now been focused on the impact of nutrition on pediatric age and disease processes. The dramatic phase of growth from birth to 18 years of age must be considered when tailoring nutritional support regimens for healthy children, as well as for those with acute and chronic disease processes.

Protein and energy must be provided to meet both the basal and growth requirements of the patient and to compensate for the increased metabolic requirements demanded by the disease. Disease-specific effects on digestion and absorption are another variable that must be entered into the equation utilized to calculate nutritional needs of sick children. Other differences considered in the pediatric population involve the child's dependency on caregivers to provide the nutrition. The input and cooperation of these caregivers is essential when formulating and implementing the nutritional regimen. In addition, the development of self-image and body image occurs during childhood and adolescence. Therefore, clinicians must recognize the impact that poor nutrition can have on these developmental processes (Yowell-Warman & Quees, 1989).

Once it has been determined that a patient is a candidate for home nutrition support, the optimal site, route, and feeding schedule need to be determined. Enteral nutrition (EN) is the preferred route and parenteral nutrition (PN) should be used only in patients who have conditions that preclude the use of the gastrointestinal tract.

Pediatric Nutritional Assessment

Identification of nutritional requirements is based on the standard pediatric nutritional assessment, including feeding skills. The patient's calorie, protein, fluid, vitamin, and mineral needs are estimated from basic guidelines (Tables 5.1-5.3)

Recommended dietary allowances are used to determine initial nutrition goals, the current nutritional status and the desired need for "catch-up" growth which must be considered. The following is a formula for estimating catch-up growth.

TABLE 5.1

Energy, Protein, and Fluid Requirements

	Age	Weight	Kcal	Protein	Fluid
	(years)	*(Kg)*	*(/Kg)*	*(gm/Kg)*	*(ml)*
Premature Infants	(26-36 wks)	2.5-6	110-150	2.0-2.5	120-160
Infants	0-.5	6	115	2.2	140-160
	.5-1.0	9	105	2.0	125-145
Children	1-3	13	100	1.8	115-125
	4-6	20	86	1.5	90-110
	7-10	28	86	1.2	70-85
Males	11-14	45	60	1.0	70-85
	15-18	42	42	.8	40-50
Females	11-14	46	48	1.0	70-85
	15-18	55	38	.8	50-60

Adapted from Recommended Dietary Allowances, Ed 9, Washington, D.C. NAS, 1980.

TABLE 5.2

RDA for vitamins and minerals in infants and children (yrs)

(M/F)	0.0-0.5	0.5-1	1-3	4-6	7-10	11-14 (M/F)	15-18 (M/F)
A (IU)	1400	1330	1330	1665	2330	3330/2660	3330/2660
D (IU)	400	400	400	400	400	400	400
E (IU)	4.5	6	7.5	9	10.5	12	15/12
C (mg)	35	35	45	45	45	50	60
Folacin (mg)	0.03	0.04	0.1	0.2	0.3	0.4	0.4
Thiamin (mg)	0.3	0.5	0.7	0.9	1.2	1.4/1.1	1.4/1.1
Riboflavin (mg)	0.4	0.6	0.8	1.0	1.4	1.6/1.3	1.7/1.3
B6 (mg)	0.3	0.6	1.0	1.1	1.4	1.7/1.4	2.0/1.5
B12 (mg)	0.3	0.5	0.7	1.0	1.4	2.0/2.0	2.0/2.0
Niacin (mg)	5	6	9	12	13	17/15	20/15
Ca^{++} (mg)	400	600	800	800	800	1200/1200	1200/1200
PO_4 (mg)	300	500	800	800	800	1200/1200	1200/1200
Mg (mg)	40	60	80	120	170	270/280	400/300
Fe (mg)	6	10	10	10	10	12/15	12/15
Zn (mg)	5	5	10	10	10	15/12	15/12

Source: Food and Nutrition Board, National Academy of Sciences–National Research Council: Recommended Dietary Allowances, 1989.

TABLE 5.3

Suggested daily parenteral infusion of trace elements for pediatrics

	< 3 kg infant and/or high stool or ostomy output	> 3 kg to 5 yrs	> 5 yrs to adult
zinc	300 mcg/kg	100 mcg/kg	2.5-4.0 mg
copper	20 mcg/kg	20 mcg/kg	0.5-1.5 mg
chromium	0.14-1.2 mcg/kg	0.14-0.2 mcg/kg	10-15 mcg
manganese	2-10 mcg/kg	2-10 mcg/kg	0.15-0.8 mg

Source: AMA Department of Foods and Nutrition: Guidelines for essential trace element preparations for parenteral use. JAMA 241 (19):2051-2054, 1979. © Copyright 1979, American Medical Association. Reprinted with permission.

Estimating energy and protein needs for catch-up growth:

$$Kcal/kg = \frac{Ideal\ Weight\ for\ Height\ x\ RDA\ (kcal/kg)\ Height\ Age}{Actual\ Weight}$$

$$Protein\ (gm/kg) = \frac{Ideal\ Weight\ for\ Height\ x\ RDA\ Protein\ (gm/kg)\ Height\ Age}{Actual\ Weight}$$

Abbreviation: RDA, recommended dietary allowances.

As caloric goals are increased, protein intake should be monitored. Nutritional status is assessed and monitored with the use of anthropometrics. Height, weight, and weight for length are compared to standard growth charts. Mid-arm muscle area is used rather than mid-arm circumference, because it is considered to be a more sensitive measure of somatic protein stores in the pediatric population.

Pediatric Nutrition

The pediatric population which would benefit from parenteral nutrition are those children with a weight loss of over 10%, individuals who fail to gain weight and children with an inability to tolerate enteral alimentation. Serum albumin levels less than 3.5 g/dl and a total lymphocyte count less than 1500/dl are significant findings.

Pediatric enteral nutrition

Once it has been determined that a patient is a candidate for home nutrition support, the optimal site, route and feeding schedule need to be chosen. Sites for provisions of nutrition support are similar to those in adults.

Enteral feedings should be started at one to two milliliters per kilogram of body weight per hour, and advanced by five to ten milliliters every 12 to 24 hours until the child's established nutrition needs are met. If the child has been unable to take anything by mouth for more than three days, the formula should be started at half strength and increased as tolerated. Do not increase volume and strength simultaneously. (Hohenbrink & Oddleifson, 1989).

Children on EN support should be seen by the nutrition team as needed until the maximum rate and strength is tolerated. A visit should be planned within one month after the maximum goal has been achieved. Factors influencing the frequency and extent of further monitoring include the patient's age, nutrition status, and medical condition, as well as the family's competence. Growth velocity, Table 5.4, is useful to detect changes in nutritional status and monitor effectiveness of nutritional regimens.

Growth suppression can occur as a result of undernutrition or illness. During the recovery phase, a child can grow at a rate greater than expected for age, so, as rapid growth proceeds, the child "catches up" to his or her growth curve. During these periods of rapid growth, more frequent adjustments to the nutrition prescription may be required. Therefore, growth should be compared to reference standards for age and the feeding regimen modified as needed.

TABLE 5.4

Growth Velocity

Age	Weight increase (grams/day)
0-3 months	25-35
3-6 months	15-21
6-12 months	10-13
1-6 years	5-8
7-10 years	5-11

Source note: Adapted from American Journal of Clinical Nutrition, Vol. 35, pp. 1169-1175, with permission of American Society for Clinical Nutrition, Inc., © 1982.

Pediatric Parenteral Nutrition

Adult and pediatric PN solutions contain the same basic nutrients: water, glucose, amino acids, lipids, electrolytes, vitamins, minerals, and trace elements. General protein guidelines for pediatric patients (Hohenbrink & Oddleifson, 1989):

1. premature infant

    (a) begin: 0.25–0.5 g/kg/d

    (b) advance: 0.5 g/kg after 1–2 days as tolerated, to goal

2. older infants and children

    (a) begin: 0.5–1.0 g/kg/d

    (b) advance: 0.5–1.0 g/kg/d as tolerated, to goal

3. teenagers

    (a) begin: 1.0 g/kg/d

    (b) advance: 1.0 g/kg/d as tolerated, to goal

Dextrose is used as the carbohydrate source and usually provides fifty to sixty percent of the non-protein calories. Dextrose concentrations for peripheral PN solutions should not exceed 10%; concentrations greater than 10% are associated with increased incidence of phlebitis. Central line infusions vary from 15% not to exceed 35%; concentrations greater than 25% may be associated with increased incidence of thrombosis (Hohenbrink & Oddleifson, 1989). To prevent glycosuria, the dextrose concentrations should be gradually increased.

Lipids are used to provide non-protein calories and essential fatty acids. Infants and children require approximately three percent of total calories (0.5–1.0 gm/kg/d) as fat to prevent essential fatty acid deficiency (EFAD).

A 20% lipid emulsion can provide twice the caloric density with only slightly higher osmolality than 10% lipid. Fat emulsions may be used in both central and peripheral PN administration. Contraindications and monitoring of lipids is similar to the adult and will be discussed in the section on adult nutritional intervention.

Parenteral nutrition (PN) must be monitored closely for metabolic abnormalities. Patients should be seen by the nutrition team weekly for the first month after initiation of PN, biweekly for the second month, and then less frequently unless complications arise (Dwyer, Baker, & Richardson, 1987). Recommendations for patient monitoring include:

- anthropometric measurements (each visit)
- assessment of the patient's transition to enteral feedings (each visit)
- biochemical indexes (each visit)
- complete blood cell count (each visit)
- liver function studies (every three months)
- evaluation for deficiencies in trace elements (yearly)
- bone age (every 6–12 months.)

Therapy directed toward demonstrating and teaching normal feeding skills should be included for children. Oral motor stimulation programs are particularly important for children younger than four years who have never acquired feeding skills. The nutrition team should ensure that an oral-motor stimulation program is in place when beginning nutrition support, even when the prospect of feeding by mouth is not imminent. Children who do not learn to associate the oral stimulation experienced during feeding with a feeling of fullness and satiety will require a great deal of oral motor and behavioral intervention while learning to eat.

Adult Nutrition Support

The primary goal of nutritional therapy for the adult cancer patient is reversal or prevention of malnutrition and maintenance of adequate nutritional status throughout the course of the primary disease. Individualization of nutrition intervention strategies is as important in implementation as in goal setting.

Once the rationale for nutritional therapy has been established and individual goals have been set, the route of administration needs to be determined. Enteral feedings should be considered for those patients who cannot, or will not, consume adequate macronutrients orally. Inadequate intake in the cancer patient is conceivable due to pain, anorexia, severe vomiting, nausea, odynophagia, partial or total obstruction, coma, or fistula in the upper gastrointestinal tract. The enteral route is preferred, when feasible, as it allows the gut to function normally, is less expensive, and has fewer risks than parenteral nutrition.

Adult Nutrition Assessment

Nutritional assessment of the adult with cancer is a difficult clinical problem. The first step in the solution to this problem is to identify the cause for the altered nutritional status. A sample nutrition screening form is shown in Table 5.5 which can help identify potential feeding problems.

Nutrient recommendations are based on knowledge of nutrition status, including pre-existing deficiencies and current requirements related to clinical status. Nutrient needs depend on the type of disease, extent of disease, and type of treatment. Cancer affects the nutritional status of the individual. The method of treatment that is employed (radiation, chemotherapy, surgery and immunotherapy) may lead to many nutritional problems as noted in Table 5.6.

TABLE 5.5

Initial Nutrition Screening Form

1. Which of the following diet restrictions are you following?

| None | Low Fat | Low Cholesterol |
| Low Sugar | Low Lactose | Low Sodium (salt) |

2. Do you have any personal food restrictions?

| None | Religious | Vegetarian | Please list: |
| Intolerances | Dislikes | Food Allergies | |

3. Where do you eat Breakfast?

| Home | Other | Prepared by Self | Other |

Where do you eat Lunch?

| Home | Other | Prepared by Self | Other |

Where do you eat Dinner?

| Home | Other | Prepared by Self | Other |

4. What kind of food consistency or texture can you tolerate at this time?

| Regular | Soft | Pureed | Liquid |

5. How is your appetite? Is it:

| Good | Better | Worse | than before your illness? |

6. Do you have any of the following problems?

| No | Yes | If yes, please check. |

Sore mouth or throat
Lack of teeth
Diarrhea
Lack of saliva-dry mouth
Feeling of fullness
Constipation
Change in taste or smell
Food aversion
Nausea
Chewing Pain
Vomiting
Swallowing
Anxiety
Effect of Therapy

7. What is your usual weight?

How tall are you?

Have you lost weight recently?   Gained weight?   How much?

Over what period of time? Why?

8. Do you take vitamins or minerals?   Yes   No
Please list completely:

9. Do you take a liquid nutritional supplement?

Example:

Table 5.6.
Cancer Treatment Effects On Nutritional Status

1. Radiation treatment

   A. Radiation of oropharyngeal area

      1) Destruction of sense of taste; xerostomia and odynophagia; loss of teeth

   B. Radiation to lower neck and mediastinum

      1) Esophagitis with dysphagia

      2) Fibrosis with esophageal stricture

   C. Radiation of abdomen and pelvis

      1) Bowel damage, acute and chronic, with diarrhea, malabsorption, stenosis and obstruction, fistulization

2. Surgical treatment

   A. Radical resection of oropharyngeal area

      1) Chewing and swallowing difficulties

   B. Esophagectomy

      1) Gastric stasis and hypochlorhydria secondary to vagotomy

      2) Steatorrhea secondary to vagotomy

      3) Diarrhea secondary to vagotomy

      4) Early satiety

      5) Regurgitation

   C. Gastrectomy (high subtotal or total)

      1) Dumping syndrome

      2) Malabsorption

      3) Achlorhydria and lack of intrinsic factor and R protein

      4) Hypoglycemia

      5) Early satiety

   D. Intestinal resection

      1) Jejunum

         a) Decreased efficiency of absorption of many nutrients

      2) Ileum

         a) Vitamin B_{12} deficiency

         b) Bile salt losses with diarrhea or steatorrhea

         c) Hyperoxaluria and renal stone

         d) Calcium and magnesium depletion

         e) Fat and fat-soluble vitamin malabsorption

Table 5.6.

Cancer Treatment Effects On Nutritional Status

(continued)

    3) Massive bowel resection
        a) Life-threatening malabsorption
        b) Malnutrition
        c) Metabolic acidosis
        d) Dehydration
    4) Ileostomy and colostomy
        a) Complications of salt and water balance
  E. Blind loop syndrome
    1) Vitamin B_{12} malabsorption
  F. Pancreatectomy
    1) Malabsorption
    2) Diabetes mellitus

3. Drug treatment
  A. Corticosteroids
    1) Fluid and electrolyte problems
    2) Nitrogen and calcium losses
    3) Hyperglycemia
  B. Sex hormone and analogues
    1) May induce nausea and vomiting
  C. Immunotherapy
    1) Interleukin-2
        a) Azotemia
        b) Hypotension
        c) Fluid retention
  D. Antimetabolites, alkylating agents, and other drugs

Source: Shills ME: Nutrition and diet in cancer. In: Shills ME, Young VR (eds): Modern Nutrition in Health and Disease. Lea & Febiger Publishers, PA. 1988. p. 1408. Reprinted with permission.

Nutritional therapy will be based on determining caloric requirements for the individual. Predicting and calculating energy requirements are often difficult. Approximations may be necessary when dealing with the patient in the homecare setting. Two methods used to predict caloric expenditure are identified below.

Harris-Benedict Equation=Resting Energy Expenditure (REE):

$66.47 + 13.75W + 5.0H - 6.76A$ (men)

$665.1 + 9.56W + 1.85H - 4.68A$ (women)

W: weight in kilograms

H: height in centimeters

A: age in years

REE x activity factor = Total energy expenditure

Activity factors: 1.2 bedridden and 1.3 ambulatory

Total Calories Per Kilogram Body Weight Per Day:

(1)–20–25 kcal/kg: non-ambulatory or sedentary

(2)–30–35 kcal/kg: slightly hypermetabolic; for weight gain/ anabolism

(3)–35 kcal/kg: hypermetabolic or severely stressed; significant malabsorption.

History of weight loss is generally considered significant to health and recovery. Some awareness of average weights for the American adult population is useful in placing the patient on a scale of depletion, adequate nourishment, or obesity. Appendix 10 provides a standard for height and weight with regards to age, sex and frame.

Protein requirements vary with age and clinical situation. The following recommendations can serve as guidelines for determination of protein needs. (Bloch, 1989)

minimal daily requirements	0.5g/kg
normal maintenance level	0.8–1.0g/kg
hypermetabolic	1.5–2.5g/kg

Fat is required because it functions as a carrier for fat-soluble vitamins, and provides essential fatty acids. It is needed as a constituent of cell membranes, as an insulating agent, as padding around vital organs, and as a rich source of energy. Essential fatty acid deficiency (EFAD) is rare in a population consuming varied foods. Patients who are unable to eat and are dependent on enteral or parenteral support, especially for weeks or months, are at higher risk for development of this condition (Lang & Schulte, 1987).

Fluid requirements depend on current medical conditions (e.g. fever, renal disease, diarrhea, and gastrointestinal fistulas), as well as normal fluid losses (insensible water loss, excretion in urine and feces). In the comatose or severely debilitated patient who is unable to consume additional water voluntarily, dehydration and hyperosmolar diuresis or diarrhea may be life threatening. Two common methods of calculating fluid requirements are shown below.

Method 1	Fluid
For young, vigorous, previously	(ml/kg)
healthy adults	40
For other adults	35
For elderly adults	30

Method 2

For the first 10 kg body weight, add 100 ml/kg/day

For the second 10 kg body weight, add 50 ml/kg/day

For each additional kg, add 20 ml/kg/day if 50 years of age or less, or add 15 ml/kg/day if older than 50

Another acceptable method is to provide 1 ml of water per calorie supplied.

That a variety of vitamins and minerals are required is accepted. However, the quantities of these nutrients needed by individuals, even in times of health, vary widely with some individuals requiring considerably higher amounts than others and some being able to manage well on very minimal quantities. The detection of minor deficiencies of either vitamins or minerals is difficult because serum levels of these nutrients are of limited value. In ensuring an adequate supply of vitamins and minerals for the ill patient, knowledge of previous dietary habits, as well as of ordinary and extraordinary needs, is helpful.

Adult Enteral Nutrition

Successful enteral therapy requires an understanding of the gastrointestinal (GI) physiology and the metabolic alterations inherent in disease processes and therapy. Using appropriate administration techniques, various solutions, and selected enteral equipment is essential to reducing the potential GI disturbances and mechanical and metabolic complications that can occur with this method of feeding. Initiation of parenteral therapy should never preclude the re-evaluation of bowel function for the possibility of enteral therapy. Evaluation of bowel function is required to initiate and continue provision of adequate nutrients by the enteral route. The options for enteral access are transnasal intubation, percutaneous endoscopic gastrostomy or jejunostomy, and surgical gastrostomy or jejunostomy. The route of access should be adapted to the patient's needs.

Product selection should take into consideration characteristics such as osmolality, viscosity, nutrient adequacy, cost, and convenience. Regardless of formula type, nutrition requirements are the most important consideration. The disease process may influence not only the patient's nutrition requirements but also the ability to digest and absorb nutrients. Elemental or predigested products may be required when malabsorption is present. Table 5.7 provides a summary of the classification of enteral tube feeding formulas and patient indicators.

TABLE 5.7

Classification of Enteral Tube Feeding Formulas

Product Category	Product Characteristics	Patient Indications	Examples of Commercial Products
Standard	• Intact macronutrients • Mimics composition of standard American diet (50%–60% carbohydrate, 10%–15% protein, 25%–40% fat calories); isomolar to blood (300 mOsm/kg)	• Fully functional gastrointestinal tract • Nothing by mouth<7 days	Isocal (Mead Johnson) Isosource (Sandoz) Fortison (Sherwood) Newtrition (Knight Medical) Nutren (Clintec) Osmolite (Ross)
High-nitrogen	• Intact macronutrients • >15% of total calorie as protein	• Malnourished • Catabolic • Elderly	Isotein HN (Sandoz) Newtrition (Knight Medical) Osmolite HN (Ross) Sustacal (Mead Johnson) Travasorb (HN) (Clintec)
Predigested/elemental	• Hydrolyzed macronutrients • Hyperosmolar (>450 mOsm/kg) • Generally low in total fat (<10%) • or may contain 30% of calories as fat with <50% from long-chain triglyceride	• Partially functioning gastrointestinal tract • Nothing by mouth >7 days	Criticare HN (Mead Johnson) Peptamen (Clintec) Reabilan (O'Brien) Vital/High Nitrogen (Ross) Vivonex T.E.N. (Norwich Eaton)
Concentrated	• Intact macronutrients • Mimics composition of typical American diet	• Restricted fluid intake	Isocal HCN (Mead Johnson) Magnacal (Sherwood) TwoCal HN (Ross)
Fiber-containing/blenderized	• Contains fiber from natural food sources or from added soy polysaccharide	• Bowel function regulation	Compleat (Sandoz) Enrich (Ross) Jevity (Ross) Vitaneed (Sherwood)
Specialty products for liver, renal, and pulmonary disease	• Varies depending on disease state	• Organ failure (renal or hepatic) or pulmonary compromise	Amin-Aid (Kendall) Hepatic Aid (Kendall) Pulmocare (Ross)

Nutritional completeness can be ensured by evaluating the product for the quantity and quality of nutrients, ratio of one nutrient component to another, and volume of solution required to meet 100% of the U.S. RDA for vitamins. The most frequently compared nutrient components are protein, fat and carbohydrate. Often the amount of a specific electrolyte contained in the enteral solution must be calculated.

The array of enteral formulas available to choose from is wide and beyond the scope of this discussion. However, nutrient analysis for a variety of enteral products can be obtained from formula manufacturers. The following is a brief summary of the classification system:

Standard Tube Feedings. Generally, they are ready to use, provide 1kcal/ml of energy and are lactose free. They consist of both simple and complex carbohydrates, intact proteins, and long and medium chain triglycerides. They have a low osmolality and viscosity, which allows easy flow of solution through a small bore tube. Usually 1.5 to 2.0 liters is required to meet the RDA for vitamins and minerals and fluid needs.

Calorically-Dense Formulas: These products are more concentrated to provide 1.5 to 2.0 kcal/ml. Patients who require fluid restrictions can benefit from products. Hydration status should be monitored closely to prevent dehydration or overfeeding.

Elemental and Predigested Formulas: These products require minimal digestion and decrease secretions into the GI tract. Therefore, patients with impaired digestive and absorptive capabilities are candidates for these solutions. They are low residue, lactose free, provide 1 kcal/ml and require 1.5 – 2.0 liters/day to meet the RDA for vitamins and minerals. The high solute and carbohydrate loads increase osmolality which may cause diarrhea and glucose intolerance. The fat content is usually 1–12 percent of total calories with inclusion of essential fatty acids.

Disease Specific Formulas: Patients with renal failure may use a product that contains a higher percent of essential amino acids. They are usually calorically dense, have a high osmolality, and low concentrations of certain electrolytes. Another product used for patients with liver failure provides higher levels of branched-chain and lower levels of aromatic, amino acids.

Once enteral feeding is chosen, formula administration is considered. Bolus feedings involve the rapid administration of 250 to 500ml of solution several times daily. Intermittent feedings may also be administered several times daily, but over at least 1/2 hour by gravity drip or controlled pump infusion. This method is better tolerated. Home patients may be able to tolerate cyclic nighttime feedings given over 8–10 hours. This allows more freedom during the day. The delivery technique and the formula selection will determine the guidelines for initiation of enteral therapy. This will need to be individualized for each patient.

Complications may be classified as GI disturbances, mechanical complications, and metabolic complications. Tables 5.8 – 5.10 list potential complications, causes and preventions regarding enteral therapy. Over time enteral feedings may produce many unique side effects. Careful monitoring of the patient is essential to prevent the occurrence of these complications.

Adult Parenteral Nutrition

Parenteral nutrition should be considered if the gut is not functioning adequately to allow normal absorption and assimilation of nutrients or if enteral nutrition support is not adequate to meet nutritional needs. Copeland (1986) noted three criteria for parenteral nutrition in the patient with cancer: (1) patients who meet criteria for malnutrition and have a reasonable chance of responding to appropriate cancer therapy; (2) patients who have been previously treated with oncologic therapy and are incapable of adequate enteral nutrition because of the malnutrition imposed by previous therapy; (3) nutritionally intact patients whose treatment plan necessitates multiple courses of chemotherapy, possibly combined with radiation therapy or surgery, when optimal nutritional status during treatment is a necessary goal.

Energy substrates commonly used in parenteral nutrition are dextrose solution and lipid emulsions. Synthetic crystalline amino acid solutions are used to provide a source of nitrogen for protein synthesis. In addition, solutions are supplemented with those vitamins and trace elements that have been determined to be essential. The route of nutrient administration, disease-specific constraints on nutrient delivery, nutritional requirements, and the goals of nutritional support influence substrate source and quantity.

The monohydrate form of dextrose provides the carbohydrate source. Each gram of dextrose monohydrate provides 3.4 kcal upon complete oxidation. The minimum amount of carbohydrate required by man is unknown, but a figure of 100 grams per day is frequently used; inadequate carbohydrate administration results in utilization of protein as an energy source. The maximum amount of carbohydrate tolerated is approximately 5mg/kg/min; excessive carbohydrate administration has been associated with synthesis and storage of fat, hepatic dysfunction, and increased CO_2 production causing respiratory failure (Skipper, 1989).

Parenteral lipid emulsions are routinely used as a source of essential fatty acids. They provide a concentrated caloric source of 9kcal/g. Essential fatty acids should comprise 4% of the caloric intake to prevent EFAD. Approximately 20–40% of non-protein calories from fat provides optimum protein sparing, and a maximum of 60% is recommended.

Crystalline or synthetic amino acid solutions contain 40—50% essential amino acids (EAA) and 50–60% nonessential amino acids (NEAA) with varying amounts of electrolytes (Louie & Niemiec, 1986). Products differ in their individual amino acid profiles as well as their available concentrations and electrolyte content. Standard base solutions

TABLE 5.8

Gastrointestinal complications associated with enteral nutrition therapy

Complication	Possible Causes	Prevention/Therapy
1. Nausea/vomiting Cramping Distention Bloating Hypermotility	• Inappropriate formula administration (i.e., rapid increase in rate/volume or rapid increase in concentration) • Lactose intolerance • Antibiotic therapy • Cold formula	• Initiate and advance formula rate and concentration gradually; reduce rate and/or concentration temporarily • Change to lactose free formula • Lactinex Rx • Bring formula to room temperature before use
2. Diarrhea	• Inappropriate formula administration • Starvation/hypoalbunemia • Antibiotic therapy • Malabsorption (Short Bowel Syndrome, Compromised Pancreatic Function, Severe Crohn's Disease, Radiation Enteritis) • Lactose Intolerance • Contaminated formula/equipment • Pellagra	• Initiate and advance formula rate and concentration gradually • Reduce rate and/or concentration temporarily • Continuous infusion administration technique • Use elemental diet initially until nutritional status improves • Lactinex granules (one packet via tube, 3 times per day for one day) • Bolus doses of pancreatic enzymes via feeding tube several times a day • Elemental diet • Lactose free formula • Change solutions and clean all equipment • 100mg nicotinamide per liter of enteral solution per day
3. High gastric residuals (gastric retention)	• Reduced gastric motility • Inactivity (bed rest)	• Elevate HOB more than 30° • Gastric stimulants • Feed into small bowel
4. Constipation	• Inadequate H_2O intake • Reduced gastric motility • Inadequate bulk • Drug Rx	• Increase free water intake • Stool softener • Fiber containing formula • Prune juice if allowed • Increase activity if possible

Adapted from:Konstantinides NN, Shronts EP. Tube feeding: Managing the basics. Am J Nurs 83(9): 1313-1323, 1983.

TABLE 5.9

Mechanical Complications associated with enteral nutrition therapy

Complication	Possible Causes	Prevention/Therapy
1. Pharyngeal irritation; Nasopharyngeal/mucosal erosion;	• Large bore vinyl or rubber feeding tubes for prolonged periods of time	• Small bore polyurethane or silicone feeding tube
2. Obstruction of the feeding tube lumen	• Particulate matter from crushed medications administered through the tube	• Thorough crushing of medications or use liquid form
	• Incompletely dissolved formula secondary to poor mixing technique	• Thorough mixing of enteral formula
	• Failure to irrigate tube	• Flushing of feeding tube after medication administration and after feedings are interrupted • Patency restored by irrigating with — warm water mixed with 1 tsp. non-potato flaked meat tenderizer, or — 1/4 tsp. pancreatic enzyme powder mixed with 15ml water
3. Aspiration; Gastric retention	• Altered gastric motility, altered gag reflex • Patient's head of bed not elevated adequately during feeding and for 2 hours after • Displaced feeding tube • Poor gastric emptying	• Continuous infusion administration • Elevate head of bed 30° or more • Monitor rube placement • Position feeding tube distal to the ligament of Treitz
4. Tube displacement	• Coughing, vomiting	• Replace tube and confirm placement by x-ray

Adapted from : Konstantinides NN, Shronts EP: Tube feeding: Managing the basics. AM J Nurs 83(9): 1313-1332, 1983.

TABLE 5.10

Metabolic complications associated with enteral nutrition therapy

Complication	Possible Causes	Prevention/Therapy
1. Glucose intolerance Hyperosmolar Hyperglycemic nonketotic dehydration/coma	• Stress (traumatic or septic) with a temporary insulin resistance • Diabetes Mellitus	• Insulin administration • Use of formula with 30-50% calories as fat • Increase free water intake
2. Hyponatremia	• Dilutional state • Excess GI losses	• Diuretic therapy • Restrict fluids
3. Hypernatremia	• Free water loss secondary to: • Diabetes Insipidus • Dehydration	• Appropriate hydration
4. Hypokalemia	• Dilutional states • Diuretic therapy • Large dose insulin therapy • Increased losses (e.g., GI drainage, diarrhea) • Refeeding syndrome in malnourished patients	• Diuretic therapy • Potassium supplementation
5. Hyperkalemia	• Metabolic acidosis secondary to renal insufficiency	• Use of enteral formula with low levels of K+
6. Hypophosphatemia	• Large dose insulin therapy • Refeeding syndrome in malnourished patients	• Phosphate supplementation
7. Hyperphosphatemia	• Renal insufficiency	• Use of enteral formula with low levels of phosphate
8. Hypozincemia	• Increased losses (e.g., GI drainage, burns, diarrhea, diuretics)	• Zinc supplementation
9. Essential fatty acid deficiency	• Use of enteral formula with low fat content over a prolonged period of time	• Provide a minimum of 4% of the caloric intake as essential fatty acids (linoleic)
10. Excess CO_2 production Respiratory insufficiency	• Overfeeding calories, especially as carbohydrate	• Provide an enteral formula with balanced CHO, PRO, FAT content • Increase % Kcal provided as fat • Do not overfeed

Adapted from: Konstantinides NN, Shronts EP: Tube feeding: Managing the basics. Am J Nurs 83 (9): 1313-1323, 1983.

for PN usually contain 500ml of 8.5% or 10% amino acids and 500ml of concentrated dextrose. Although protein has a caloric value of 4.0 kcal/g if oxidized, the amino acids are not calculated as a calorie source in paren-

TABLE 5.II

Electrolytes in TPN Solutions

Electrolyte	Daily Requirement
Sodium	60–150 mmol
Potassium	70–150 mmol
Chloride	60–150 mmol
Magnesium	0.35–0.45 mEq/kg/body weight
Calcium	0.2–0.3 mEq/kg/body weight
Phosphate	7–10 mmol/1000 kcal

Source: Reprinted from Handbook of Total Parenteral Nutrition by J.P. Grant, p. 98, with permission of W.B. Saunders Company, Philadelphia, © 1980.

teral solutions. For normal individuals, about 300 calories is needed to spare one gram of nitrogen, but in critical illness, about 100–150 calories is needed.

Parenteral vitamin requirements differ from enteral vitamin requirements due to differences in efficiency of absorption and utilization of nutrients administered via the enteral and parenteral routes.

The six major electrolytes are sodium, potassium, magnesium, calcium, phosphate, and chloride, all of which have an active role in the metabolic processes of the body. When refeeding severely malnourished patients or when using high levels of dextrose in the PN formulation, the requirement for the intracellular electrolytes (potassium, phosphate and magnesium) increases. The electrolyte content is dependent on individual patient requirements.

Other additives that need to be considered are Vitamin K, which can be added once a week; heparin, 1000 units/liter, to minimize vein thrombosis; and insulin is included to control serum glucose levels during infusion. Glucose levels should remain below 200 mg/100ml during the infusion. Fat emulsions can be given 2–3 times weekly through a separate line, or a three-in-one admixture can be used. It involves the addition of the fat emulsion to the primary nutrient mixture, which is usually recommended for home patients.

The optimum administration schedule is one that minimizes the number of hours required to complete the infusion and is compatible enough with the patient's lifestyle to promote compliance. Night-time schedules for infusion may be preferred so as not to interfere with daytime activities. Usually an 8 to 16 hour cyclic infusion is tolerated and allows the patient more freedom.

Regardless of the method of initial nutrient need determination, patients require periodic assessment to avoid the complications of both over and underfeeding. Baseline triglyceride levels are important to determine pre-existing hyperlipidemia. Serum triglyceride concentrations respond dramatically to the infusion rate of lipid emulsions. Clearance of lipid emulsions is most commonly assessed by plasma triglyceride concentration 6–8 hours following cessation of fat infusion. Upper limits for triglyceride are usually 250mg/dl during a continuous infusion for children and 300–350mg/dl 6 hours post infusion for adults.

Glucose intolerance is among the most common complications of PN. It may occur when large glucose doses are initiated too quickly, or during stress. Providing a greater proportion of calories as fat may be beneficial for patients with impaired insulin response.

CONCLUSION

Cancer patients are frequently malnourished at the time of diagnosis. These patients develop anorexia and reduced nutritional intake. Specific abnormalities in substrate metabolism and energy expenditure have been detected. There is little doubt that malnutrition associated with cancer has a negative prognostic effect and can contribute directly to the demise of the patient as well as increase postoperative morbidity.

Nutritional therapy is an important supportive measure. In the future, more specific manipulation of substrates and hormones administered to the host may provide improved results. Clinical trials of arginine supplementation to enteral feeding have shown rapid return of lymphocyte proliferation to normal following an operation.

Use of glutamine supplementation in PN may reduce the stomatitis and enteritis associated with multidrug chemotherapy. Finally, use of growth hormone or tumor necrosis factor antibodies may beneficially affect the metabolism of endogenous and exogenous substrates. (Daly, 1990).

New strategies designed to reverse cancer anorexia can pursue two goals: symptomatic care and improved nutrition. The use of the progestational agent, megestrol acetate resulted in marked increase in appetite and weight in patients with cancer. The mechanism of action of megestrol acetate is under study and it probably consists of both behavioral and metabolic effects. The action of megestrol acetate is complex involving a variety of different and interrelated target sites. Understanding these effects may help clarify underlying mechanisms of anorexia and cachexia and also provide clues for additional pharmacologic strategies. Recent studies of cytosines as mediators of anorexia and cachexia open the door to the number of potential therapeutic strategies that focus on the etiology of cancer-related undernutrition. These developments coupled with recent advances in biomedical research may well result in therapies that restore normality, not by way of forced feeding, but by antagonizing or reversing the metabolic and behavioral side effects of cancer and its treatment (Tchekmedyian, 1992).

REFERENCES

American Medical Association. (1979). Guidelines for essential trace element preparations for parenteral use. *JAMA, 241* (19): 2051–2054.

Bloch, A. (1989). Nutrition support in cancer. In E.P. Shronts (Ed.), *Nutrition Support Dietetics* (pp. 97–106). Silver Springs, MD: American Society for Parenteral and Enteral Nutrition.

Copeland, E. (1986). Intravenous hyperalimentation and cancer: a historical perspective. *Journal of Parenteral and Enteral Nutrition.* 10, 337–342.

Copeland, E.M., & Souba, W.W. (1988). Nutritional considerations in treatment of the cancer patient. *Nutrition in Clinical Practice,* 3 (5), 173–174.

Daly, J.M., Hoffman, K.H., Lieberman, M., Leon, P., Redmond, H.P., & Shou, J. (1990). Nutritional support in the cancer patient. *Journal of Parenteral and Enteral Nutrition, 14* (Suppl.5) 244S–248S.

DeWys, W. (1985). Management of cancer cachexia. *Oncology, 12,* 452–460.

Douglass H. (1984). Nutrition support of the cancer patient. *Hospital Forum, 19,* 220.

Dwyer, E., Baker, S. & Richardson, D. (1987). Home parenteral nutrition. In J. Stephen & W. Deitz (Ed), *Pediatric Nutrition Theory & Practice* (pp. 763–769). Woburn, MA: Butterworth.

Fomon, S. (1974). *Infant Nutrition* (2nd ed). Philadelphia: W.B. Saunders.

Grant, J.P. (1980). Handbook of Total Parenteral Nutrition. Philadelphia: W.B. Saunders.

Hohenbrink, K. & Oddleifson, N. (1989). Pediatric nutrition support. In E.P. Shronts (Ed.), *Nutrition Support Dietetics* (pp. 231–272). Silver Springs, MD: American Society for Parenteral and Enteral Nutrition.

Kerner, J.A. (1983). *Manual of Pediatric Parenteral Nutrition.* (pp.202–221).

Konstantinides, N.N., Shronts, E.P. (1983). Tube feeding: Managing the basics. *American Journal of Nursing, 83* (9): 1313–1323.

Lang, C.E. & Schulte, C.V. (1987). The adult patient. In C.E. Lang (Ed.), *Nutritional Support In Critical Care* (pp. 61–89). Rockville, MD: Aspen Publications.

Lenssen, P. (1989). Monitoring and complications of parenteral nutrition. In A. Skipper (Ed.), *Dietitian's Handbook of Enteral and Parenteral Nutrition* (pp. 347–373). Rockville, MD: Aspen Publications.

Louie, N. & Niemiec, P.W. (1986). Parenteral nutrition solutions. In J.L. Rombeau & M.D. Caldwell (Eds.), *Parenteral Nutrition* (pp. 272–305). Philadelphia: W.B. Saunders Co.

Palac B. (1985). Interdepartmental care for the oncology patient. *Nutritional Support Services, 5(1),* 48–51.

Shills, M.E. (1988) Nutrition and diet in cancer. In M.E. Shills, V.E. Young (Ed.), *Modern Nutrition in Health and Disease.* Philadelphia: Lea & Febiger.

Skipper, A. (1989). Parenteral nutrition. In E.P. Shronts (Ed.), *Nutrition Support Dietetics* (pp. 83—96). Silver Springs, MD: American Society for Parenteral and Enteral Nutrition.

Tchekmedyian, W.S. (1992). Evaluation of the benefits of nutritional support and new pharmacological strategies. Symposium conducted at the meeting of the Amercan Society for Parenteral and Enteral Nutrition, Orlando, FL, (February).

Wachsman, B.A. & Hardin, T.C. (1988). Cancer cachexia: the metabolic alterations. *Nutrition in Clinical Practice, 3* (5), 191–197.

Yowell-Warman, K. & Queen, P. (1989). Pediatric nutrition in the home. In M. Hermann-Zaidins & R. Touger-Decker (Eds.), *Nutrition Support in Home Health* (pp. 142–174). Rockville, MD: Aspen Publishers.

CANCER PAIN MANAGEMENT

Carol J. Swenson, RN, MS, OCN
Oncology Clinical Nurse Specialist
Swedish American Hospital, Rockford, Illinois

CANCER PAIN MANAGEMENT

Carol J. Swenson, RN, MS, OCN
Oncology Clinical Nurse Specialist
Swedish American Hospital, Rockford, Illinois

Pain has an element of blank; It cannot recollect
When it began, or if there were
A day when it was not.
— *Emily Dickinson*
"Pain Has an Element of Blank"

INTRODUCTION

Nurses play a major role in the management of the person who is experiencing cancer pain. One of the Position Statements on Cancer Pain which Spross, McGuire & Schmitt (1990) identify in the Oncology Nursing Society (ONS) Position Paper on Cancer is that "Nurses are responsible and accountable for implementation and coordination of the plan for management of cancer pain" (p.596). In the home-setting, this is most important. The nurse is the professional person who conducts the assessment of pain on an on-going basis and can most accurately determine whether the pain has increased, whether side effects are being managed adequately and, whether the client and family are satisfied with the pain relief provided.

It has been well documented that there has been a lack of professional health care education regarding pain management which has resulted in less than optimal pain management for the person with cancer (Marks & Sachar, 1973; Cohen, 1980; Watt-Watson, 1987). McCaffery & Beebe (1989) describe health professionals as often unaware of their lack of knowledge about pain control. The medications and technology are available for managing 95% of all cancer pain. Misconceptions also exist about narcotic regulations both nationally and within many states, which promote the limitation of narcotics from being prescribed even when they are needed for successful pain management.

Additionally, the lay public has many myths which are beginning to be addressed. Some of these myths include:

- the person taking pain medications will easily become addicted

- cancer pain cannot be relieved anyway; it's part of the disease

- the "strong stuff" must be saved for later when the pain gets "really bad" or else nothing will be available

- "shots" are stronger than pills

THE CANCER PAIN PROBLEM TODAY

Not all people with cancer experience pain. The incidence of cancer pain is difficult to determine, but several experts (Brescia, 1987; Bonica, 1987; Foley, 1987; Portenoy, 1989; and Weissman, Burchman, Dinndorf & Dahl, 1990) agree with the range of 50–80%. Whether pain occurs in cancer is dependent upon several factors. These factors include:

Location of the primary or metastatic site of cancer

If there is bony involvement (as occurs with spinal metastases) or neural involvement (by direct tumor invasion or compression of any nerve tissue) the pain will be more severe than when there is 'pressure' due to organ involvement.

Stage of the tumor activity

The person in a later stage of cancer experiences pain more often and of a more severe intensity than a person who is in an early stage of disease.

DEFINITIONS OF PAIN

"Whatever the experiencing person says it is, existing whenever the experiencing person says it does" (McCaffery, 1968) is the most global and client-centered definition of pain. The American Pain Society (1989) and the ONS Position Paper on Pain (1990) describe pain as "an unpleasant sensory and emotional experience associated with actual or potential tissue damage, or described in terms of such damage". From these two descriptions of pain it becomes apparent that pain is multidimensional and subjective. Two ways pain can be categorized are:

Acute Pain: brief duration (less than six months); the cause of which usually is known; the intensity may range from mild to severe.

Chronic Pain: extends beyond six months; the cause may or may not be known; it has not responded to treatment and/or does not subside after injury heals; the intensity may range from mild to severe.

Cancer Pain may be:

- both *chronic and acute*

    There is the time element of chronic pain (extending beyond six months) and yet the intensity may be severe and the pain can be described as 'intractable'

- due to *several etiologies; Tumor activity* involving bone, nerves, viscera or soft tissue

Somatic pain (nociceptive) — results from stimulation of afferent nerves in the skin, connective tissue, muscles, joints or bones. Usually described as *"dull, sharp or aching"* and is localized; the response to analgesics is usually good.

Visceral pain — involves organs in the thoracic or abdominal area. Can be caused by infiltration, pressure or distention. Pain is described as *"constant, aching, or deep"*. This type of pain may be referred to surface areas.

Visceral pain may be seen in advanced pancreatic or liver cancer. The response to analgesics is usually good.

Neuropathic pain (deafferentation) — results from peripheral or central nerve injury. Usually described as *"burning, shooting or tingling"*. Response to analgesics is usually poor.

CANCER PAIN SYNDROMES

A pain syndrome may have different types of pain, different etiologies of pain and different methods of treatment.

Some of the known pain syndromes due to direct tumor involvement are:

Bone involvement — multiple bony metastases are by far the most common cause of generalized bone pain, according to Portenoy (1989). In the case of vertebral involvement, it is imperative that the nurse report this occurrence. Pain alone will precede nerve compression and prompt intervention may prevent neurological deficit formation.

Peripheral nerves — sites where this may occur include the chest wall and retroperitoneal space which may produce pain in the back, abdomen or legs.

Brachial plexus — usually results from a primary lung tumor (Pancoast's syndrome) and there is aching in the shoulder and upper back. According to Portenoy (1989) up to 50% of clients with Pancoast syndrome will go on to develop cord compression if left untreated. It is imperative that pain is assessed thoroughly, reported accurately and treated promptly!

Epidural spinal cord compression — over 95% of patients with epidural spinal cord compression report pain, which may be focal or referred (Portenoy, 1989). The pain will precede any sensory or motor deficit. It is mandatory that any new back pain be communicated immediately to the physician.

Cancer Treatment — e.g., surgery, radiation therapy, chemotherapy may exacerbate pain.

Some of the syndromes which may follow cancer treatment include:

Postthoracotomy pain syndrome — the intercostal nerve may be damaged at the time of surgery. Usually described as a burning pain (neuropathic).

Postmastectomy pain syndrome — the intercostobrachial nerve may be damaged at the time of surgery. Usually described as a burning pain (neuropathic) and may occur soon after surgery or months later.

Postamputation syndrome — may be due to the formation of a neuroma and have lancinating (shooting) and burning components or be a phantom sensation which exhibits both continuous dysesthesias and shooting pain (Portenoy, 1989).

Multiple neural involvement — several neural areas are affected by chemotherapy (principally the vinca alkaloids [e.g., vincristine] or cis-platinum). This paraesthesia or dysesthesia tends to be dose-related and will generally improve over 6–12 months.

Mucositis — inflammation of the oral mucosa, a side effect of some chemotherapeutic agents, can produce intensely painful ulcerations. It is not uncommon for patients to require opioids to relieve pain during this period of time.

Postradiation pain — inadvertent damage to the spinal cord, mucosa or bone.

Some pains are Unrelated to cancer - (e.g., arthritis, decubitus, tension headache, diabetic neuropathy, etc.).

The immunocompromised patient may develop herpes zoster (Shingles). Following the treatment and healing phase, postherpetic neuralgia may remain. It can be difficult to manage and needs to be addressed as a neuropathic pain in origin.

Any pain has special significance for the client with cancer. Whether it is a "routine" headache or gastritis, the fear is that the pain represents an extension of the cancer. All reports of pain must be evaluated.

DRUG TOLERANCE VS. DRUG ADDICTION

Drug tolerance is the need for increasing doses of analgesic to achieve the same level of pain relief. The actual incidence of tolerance is not known and many people never develop it. When an increase of medication is required, it is more often an event of disease progression but tolerance must be considered. With drug tolerance, there is a decreased duration of relief, followed by decreased level of pain relief. If tolerance is suspected, the person can be switched to another opioid. When switching to another opioid, use one-half of the equianalgesic dose; cross-tolerance between narcotics is incomplete and the person may otherwise be overmedicated (APS, 1989).

Drug addiction is the use of narcotics for the psychological euphoric effect and not for the analgesic effect. There is overwhelming involvement with obtaining and using drugs for other than approved medical reasons. Addiction as a result of medically prescribed narcotics is rare (<1:1000). Porter & Jick (1980) report that of 11,882 hospitalized patients who received at least one opioid injection during hospitalization there were only 4 cases of documented addiction in patients with no previous history of addiction. Often health care professionals overestimate the incidence of addiction following prescribed narcotics for medical purposes. Lay public are often frightened of addiction occuring and need assurance of the appropriate use of narcotics and that addiction is a nonissue in cancer pain management.

Physical dependence is the body's adaptation to the use of narcotics without which abstinence syndrome (or withdrawal symptoms), will occur based on physiological changes. The person with cancer who is on narcotics for longer than three weeks may be physically dependent, but is not addicted.
(See page 142 - weaning the person from opioids)

NURSES' RESPONSIBILITIES RELATED TO PAIN MANAGEMENT

Although the care of patients with pain is multidisciplinary, in most cases nursing care is the cornerstone. (McCaffery, 1989).

Assessment of the Cancer Patient Experiencing Pain

Nursing is involved in obtaining a detailed quantitative and qualitative assessment of the client's pain experience. Pain is a subjective experience and it is only the person who has the pain who is able to legitimately describe the event in detail. Qualitative assessment includes the nurses' observations of behavior and appearance, the client's description of sensations and personal impact of pain. Quantitative assessment is the client description of the intensity of pain and the analgesic requirements over time.

Table 6.1 illustrates both qualitative and quantitative factors involved in pain assessment.

Appendices 5 and 6 include clinically relevant pain assessment tools.

Table 6.1

Qualitative Assessment includes:

Reported Symptoms Associated with Moderate to Severe Pain

- Mood disturbances: anxiety, depression, anger, and irritability
- Decreased ability to concentrate/communicate
- Loss of appetite, nausea, and vomiting
- Sleep disturbance/sleep deprivation
- Sexual dysfunction/lack of interest
- Splinting, limited mobility, disuse syndromes
- Fatigue
- Behavioral changes

Classification of Pain

Acute — <6 months

Chronic — >6 months

- Does the pain interfere with Activities of Daily Living (ADLs), sleep patterns (awakens due to the pain), or sociability (visiting with others, talking)?

Location

- Is it confined to one area or does it radiate?
- Has it changed from a previous location or extended beyond a previous site?

Quality

- Because the source of pain can vary, it is imperative that the nurse elicit a description which describes the pain most accurately. Use the client's own words for what the pain feels like. Keep in mind that the following descriptions may indicate a particular type of pain:

Burning — possibly neuropathic pain

Stabbing — possibly neuropathic pain

Dull, sharp, or aching — possibly somatic pain

Constant or deep — possibly visceral pain

Duration

- Onset — When did it start?
- Intermittent — Does it last briefly after movement?

- Constant — Does it never go away?
- Aggravating and relieving factors
  What makes the pain worse? …better?
  Does it help to lie down, stand, sit up?
- What has person tried?
  Analgesics?
              Type?
              Dose?
              Frequency?
  Positioning
  Heat/Cold
  Massage
- What is the expectation for pain relief?
  An acceptable level which is tolerable
  No pain

Quantitative Assessment includes:

Intensity of Pain

- 0–10 with 0 being 'no pain' and '10' the worst pain
  imaginable. A conversion of numbers into word descriptors for the
  levels may include:

  0 = None

  2 = Mild — pain unnoticed with activity

  4 = Discomforting — sometimes interferes with activities
      or sleep

  6 = Distressing — usually interferes with activities or sleep

  8 = Severe — severely "restricts" person

  10 = Excruciating — unable to tolerate

Equianalgesic amounts per 24 hours

It is important for the nurse to calculate what the total amount of
analgesics required per 24 hours has been and convert this into the
common language of morphine equivalents.

Nursing Diagnoses Associated with Cancer Pain

Spross, et al, (1990) outline the next step in the nursing process. After assessment, when caring for the person with cancer pain, nursing diagnoses are identified. Appropriate nursing diagnoses may include:

Alterations in:
- Comfort (pain, sleep and/or pruritis)
- Mobility
- Coping
- Elimination (constipation or diarrhea)
- Protective Mechanisms (e.g., risk of spinal cord compression)
- Home management
- Knowledge deficit (e.g., action of analgesics, schedule of administration, potential side effects)
- Anxiety
- Fear
- Fatigue
- Spiritual distress
- Social isolation/changes in relationships
- Hopelessness

Planning of Care for the Person in Pain

Planning follows the identification of nursing diagnoses and builds on the knowledge gained with the assessment of the patient by the nurse. In the home, the client/family must understand and agree to the current treatment plan. The client must be satisfied with the pain relief. The client must be able to tell the family and the nurse if the current plan is not relieving the pain, so additional orders can be obtained.

Pharmacologic Interventions

General Principles of Analgesic Administration

Choose the analgesic appropriate to the type of pain and the level of pain. The choice of a non-opioid or weak, or strong opioid should be based on pain intensity determined through assessment. Choice of the easiest and most cost-effective route of administration is the strategy for pain management.

The Kissing principle (Keep It Sanely Simple in Narcotic Giving) is to use the oral route whenever possible. If nausea and/or vomiting prohibit this route, try the rectal route. Consider the following progression of routes:

- Oral
- Rectal
- Transdermal
- Subcutaneous
- Intramuscular (if occasional need)
- Intravenous
- Intraspinal (epidural or intrathecal)

Schedule Administration for Around The Clock (ATC) dosing.

This is mandatory to achieve a steady-state of analgesia. Never use a PRN schedule; the pain level then escalates and the client must spend time just to "catch up" to prior levels of analgesia. The important feature is to stay ahead of the pain. This principle requires teaching and reinforcement by nurses as it differs from usual pain management to which clients are accustomed.

Whatever the medication, route or frequency of administration, always make certain that there is an order available for "breakthrough" pain. This is a sudden, and sometimes brief, increase in pain which may be due to increased activity or a particular motion. This "rescue dose" is administered over and above the regularly scheduled ATC medication. If 3–4 doses are required each 24 hours, the ATC regularly scheduled doses should be increased to include the amount used for previous breakthrough pain while still maintaining a PRN dose for future breakthrough pain.

Plan for treatment of side effects. Management of side effects must be done aggressively and often should be prophylactic. Be aware that the following side effects may occur with the repeated administration of opioids.

- Constipation (does not decrease over time)
- Nausea/Vomiting (usually temporary lasting about one week)
- Sedation (usually temporary)
- Respiratory Depression (rarely occurs)
- Other: confusion/hallucinations
      dizziness
      urinary retention

Never use placebos. Placebos have no place in the oncology client population. As McCaffrey states "pain is whatever the client says it is, whenever he says it does".

World Health Organization (WHO) Stepladder of Pain Management
The concept of an orderly progression from the occurrence of pain to its successful management can be visualized as the rungs of a ladder in the following sequence:

1. Pain exists
2. Use a non-opioid with or without an adjuvant drug
3. If pain persists or increases,
4. Use a weak opioid, with or without a non-opioid, and with or without an adjuvant drug
5. If pain persists or increases,
6. Use a strong opioid, with or without a non-opioid, and with or without an adjuvant drug

The goal of this ladder is freedom from cancer pain. Orderly progression allows for trials of various medications at all levels and assures that everything is being attempted to control the pain across the spectrum.

Non-Opioid Analgesics

Non-opioid analgesics work primarily on the peripheral nervous system. Table 6.2 gives examples of these medications. They are used for mild to moderate pain especially of bone metastases, soft-tissue infiltration, and arthritis.

TABLE 6.2

Examples of Non-Opioid Analgesics

Generic name	Trade name	Manufacturer	Usual Dose
Acetylated Salicylates:			
acetylsalicylic acid			
(aspirin)	Alka-Seltzer	Miles	650 mg q4h
	Anacin	Whitehall	
	Bufferin	Bristol-Myers	
	Equagesic	Wyeth-Ayerst	
	Norgesic	3M Riker	
Para-Aminophenol Derivatives:			
acetaminophen	Anacin-3	Whitehall	650 mg q4h
	Datril	Bristol-Myers	
	Excedrin	Bristol-Myers	
	Midol	Glenbrook	
	Panadol	Glenbrook	
	Sine-Aid	McNeil	
	Tylenol	McNeil	
acetaminophen + aspirin:	Excedrin	Bristol-Myers	
	Vanquish	Glenbrook	
Nonacetylated Salicylates:			
choline magnesium trisalicylates	Trilisate	Purdue Frederick	1500 mg q8–12h
diflunisal	Dolobid	Merck	500 mg q8–12h
salsalate	Disalcid	3M Riker	1000 mg q8–12h
	Salsitab	Upsher-Smith	1000 mg q8–12h

Generic name	Trade name	Manufacturer	Usual Dose
Proprionic Acid Derivatives:			
ibuprofen	Advil	Whitehall	200–400 mg q4–8h
	Medipren	McNeil	200–400 mg q4–8h
	Mido 200	Glenbrook	200–400 mg q4–8h
	Motrin	Upjohn	200–400 mg q4–8h
	Nuprin	Bristol-Myers	200–400 mg q4–8h
fenoprofen	Nalfon	Dista	200 mg q4–6h
fenofen calcium		Lederle; Squibb	200–400 mg q6–8h
ketoprofen	Orudis	Wyeth-Ayerst	25–50 mg q6–8h
naproxen	Naprosyn	Syntex	500 mg q8–12h
naproxen sodium	Anaprox	Syntex	275 mg q6– 8h
Indole Acetic Acid Derivatives:			
indomethacin	Indocin	Merck	50 mg q6-8h
sulindac	Clinoril	Merck	150 mg q812h
tolmetin	Tolectin	McNeil	200 mg q6–8h
Oxicam:			
piroxicam	Feldene	Pfizer	10–30 mg q–6h

Pyrrolo-pyrolle:
ketorolac (Toradol) — new injectable 30 mg q6h (should be available in oral form during 1992)

Most nonsteroidal drugs have potential gastrointestinal side effects and these side effects may limit use over time. Inturrisi (1989) and Wilke (1990) note that all NSAIDS except choline magnesium trisalicylate (Trilisate) will interfere with platelet aggregation and therefore, may not be appropriate for someone who is thrombocytopenic.

Opioid Analgesics

Opioid analgesics work primarily at the central nervous system (CNS) level. Weak opioids are used for mild to moderate pain. Table 6.3 lists opioid analgesics currently used in treatments of cancer pain. There is no ceiling effect of morphine which means that the dose can continue to be escalated to provide analgesia with increased pain levels. For some drugs there is a ceiling which means that beyond a certain dose there is no added analgesic benefit. There are exceptional instances where clients may require 1,000 mg–2,000 mg or even more per 24 hours and the person will be alert, ambulatory and participating in activities of daily living.

TABLE 6.3

Opioid Analgesics

"Weak" Opioids	Usual dose:
Codeine	30 mg q4h
Propoxyphene hydrochloride (Darvon)	65 mg q4h
Oxycodone (Roxicodone) hydrochloride	5 mg q4h
Roxicet (oxycodone 5 mg + acetaminophen 325 mg)	q4h
Tylox (oxycodone 5 mg + acetaminophen 500 mg)	q4h
Percocet (oxycodone 5 mg + acetaminophen 325 mg)	q4h
Percodan (oxycodone 5 mg + aspirin 325 mg)	q4h
Vicodin (hydrocodone bitartrate 5 mg + acetaminophen 500 mg)	q4h

"Strong" Opioid Agonists	10 mg morphine equivalents:
Morphine Sulfate	10.0 mg
Hydromorphone (Dilaudid)	1.5 mg
Levorphanol tartrate (Levo-Dromoran)	2.0 mg
Methadone (Dolophine Hydrochloride)	10.0 mg
Fentanyl (Sublimaze) (Duragesic patch)	.1 mg
Oxymorphone hydrochloride (Nurmorphan)	1.5 mg
Meperidine (Demerol)	50-100 mg

Caution on the use of Demerol for cancer pain: Meperidine (Demerol) should never be used on a continuous basis for cancer pain treatment. The metabolite (normeperidine) is a central nervous system stimulator (Kaiko, Foley, Grabinski, et al, 1983) and this can lead to tremors or seizure activity with repeated dosing.

There is a fallacy about heroin for cancer pain. The question of heroin's efficacy over morphine has been studied in detail. The conclusion is that heroin does not offer any advantage over morphine when an equianalgesic conversion is done (Kaiko, 1985 and Twycross & Lack, 1989). Heroin (diamorphine) is metabolized to morphine before it reaches the opiate receptors of the brain. Heroin was most often the narcotic of choice in the Brompton's Cocktail in hospice programs in England; now oral morphine is routinely used.

Mixed agonist-antagonists may be used in pain management. The following list is an example of these agents:

	10 mg morphine equivalents
nalbuphine (Nubain)	10 mg
butorphanol (Stadol)	2 mg
pentazocine (Talwin)	60 mg
buprenophine (Buprenex)	0.4 mg

Be cautious in using mixed agonist-antagonists. After using agonists (e.g., morphine), withdrawal-like symptoms can be precipitated when a mixed agonist-antagonist is given. If given with an agonist, the mixed form will antagonize and give poor pain relief with possible increase in psychomimetic effects.

Dosing

Most often an increasing need for medication is indicative of progressive disease or a developing complication and aggressive therapy is warranted. When it is determined that more medication is needed to manage an individual's pain, the safe plan of increasing the dose is: increase 25–50% of the previous dose.

Example: current dose: 60 mg PO morphine q4h add: 15–30 mg PO morphine q4h. Continued assessment determines whether additional increases are needed.

Obtain an order for immediate release analgesic to use for break-through pain. This dose should equal 33–50% of the regularly scheduled dose. If ≥3 rescue doses are required per 24 hours, then obtain an order which includes that amount in the ATC dosing. Do maintain the order for rescue dosing.

Abstinence (Withdrawal) Syndrome

If a person's pain decreases (e.g., following palliative radiation to bone metastases, or a nerve block being done), the opioid requirements may indeed decrease dramatically. According to the American Hospital Formulary Service (1991), abstinence syndrome (withdrawal) will occur in a mild form if someone has required $\geq$ 80 mg of morphine per day and in a severe form if $\geq$ 240 mg of morphine per day for a period of more than 30 days.

Signs & Symptoms of Withdrawal during the first 24 hours include:

- restlessness
- perspiration
- lacrimation
- gooseflesh
- rhinorrhea
- restless sleep
- yawning
- mydriasis

Signs & Symptoms of Withdrawal during 24–72 hours include:

- twitching/muscular spasms
- kicking movements
- severe aches in back, abdomen and legs
- nausea, vomiting, diarrhea
- coryza & severe sneezing
- increase in all vital signs (T,P, BP & R)

To safely "wean" the person from opioids and prevent abstinence syndrome from occurring the following formula is used: Give 25% of the previous order; decrease q48h until <10 mg (parenteral morphine equivalent) per 24 hours are given.

Example: client has been receiving 1000 mg morphine sulfate PO/24 hours (at a 3:1 ratio this is 333 mg parenteral morphine per 24 hours)

Day 1 & 2 – 250 mg PO morphine sulfate/24 hours

Day 3 & 4 – 60 mg PO morphine sulfate/24 hours

Day 5 & 6 – 15 mg PO morphine sulfate/24 hours
(this is 5 mg parenteral morphine equivalent)

Day 7 – nothing

Duration of Opioids

Be aware that not all opioids have the same duration of effectiveness. Some opioids are short-acting, some are long-acting and others fall somewhere in the middle. Scheduling must be according to how long the medication is actually lasting or the result will be pain. Table 6.4 gives duration of opioids.

TABLE 6.4

Duration of Opioids

Short-acting

fentanyl citrate injection (Sublimaze)	1/2 hr

Intermediate-acting

meperidine (Demerol)	2–4 hr
morphine	3–4 hr
hydromorphone (Dilaudid)	"
codeine	"
oxycodone	"
propoxyphene (Darvon)	"

Long-acting

methadone (Dolophine)	6–8 hr
levorphanol (Levodromoran)	"

Equianalgesia is the conversion of one route to another or from one opioid to another in an equivalent amount. When converting from one route of administration to another or from one opioid to another, it must be done in such a manner as to not undermedicate or overmedicate the client. This concept is just beginning to be realized and nurses can do much to educate other health care professionals in the process of equianalgesic conversion. Appendix 4 contains equianalgesic information.

Adjuvant (Co-analgesic) Drugs

There are several medications which have been found to be analgesic for particular types of pain and these drugs may be ordered for other than their usual indication.

Antidepressants can produce analgesia in particular circumstances and are appropriate despite a lack of emotional depression. They seem to act by increasing the serotonin level according to Cleeland, 1989. Indications for antidepressants are neuropathic pain (especially burning), depression, and insomnia. Some examples are:

nortriptyline (Pamelor)	25 mg HS
desipramine (Norpramin)	25 mg HS
imipramine (Tofranil)	25 mg HS
doxepin (Sinequan)	25 mg BID
amitryptyline (Elavil)	25 mg HS

The analgesic therapeutic dose of antidepressants is only 1/8 to 1/6 of the dose required to treat clinical depression.

Anticonvulsants are indicated in neuropathic pain especially shooting or stabbing, lancinating pains, e.g., post herpetic pain, tics, and myoclonic jerks. Some examples are carbamazepine (Tegretol) 100–200 mg/day and phenytoin (Dilantin) 3–5 mg/kg/day.

Stimulants are indicated when analgesia needs to be increased. The use of stimulants produces a reduction of the sedative effect of opioids.

Three examples of stimulants include:

- caffeine   65 mg
- dextroamphetamine   2.5–7.5 mg BID
  (Dexedrine)   (APS, 1989, e.g. 2.5 mg
                                            a.m. & noon)
- methylphenidate (Ritalin)   15 mg/day
                                            (e.g. 10 mg 8 a.m.
                                            & 5 mg noon)

Note: tolerance may develop within one month and the dose will need to be escalated, Bruera, Brenneis, Paterson & MacDonald, 1989.

Glucocorticosteroids are indicated with acute nerve compression, increased intracranial pressure, anorexia, and with mood disorders. Three glucocorticosteroids used for pain management are:

- dexamethasone (Decadron)   4–16 mg/day
  cord compression   16–96 mg/day
                                            (APS, 1989),
- methylprednisolone (Medrol) 16 mg TID, and
- prednisone   20–80 mg/day

A word of caution regarding "potentiators" to increase the effectiveness of an analgesic. Both medicine and nursing have long taught that when the phenothiazine promethazine (Phenergan) is added to a narcotic, it will intensify (or potentiate) the analgesic effect of the narcotic. Studies by McGee and Alexander (1979) and Dundee and Moore (1961) show that in fact promethazine may increase the awareness of one's pain. McCaffery calls this an antianalgesic effect. What is observed is a potentiation of the side effects: increased sedation, hypotention and respiratory depression. The American Pain Society (1989) states that "except for methotrimeprazine [Levoprome 10–20 mg. available in parenteral formulation only], phenothiazines neither relieve pain nor potentiate opioid analgesia" (p 22).

ROUTES OF ADMINISTRATION

Oral is the route of choice for economy, safety and long duration of management. Severe pain requiring high doses of narcotics can be managed orally as long as the client is able to swallow medication without difficulty. It is important to convert the parenteral to oral doses correctly.

They are different preparations and amounts cannot be interchanged. Teach the client/family that "shots" are not necessary to control pain and that parenteral administration does not mean stronger medication. Provided the equianalgesic amount is the same, the analgesic effect will be the same. Sustained release morphine is now available which makes 12-hour dosing a possibility.

The buccal or sublingual surface may be used for absorption of liquid analgesics in small quantities.

If oral administration is not possible due to nausea/vomiting or if the person is unable to swallow or if there is fear of injections, the same dose of oral medication administered rectally can also achieve pain relief. Controlled studies are not available to support the practice fully, but it appears that the rectal mucous membrane absorbs equally to the oral cavity. Use of a rectal route may prevent the necessity of changing to a parenteral route. The limitations for this route include the presence of diarrhea, anal/rectal fissures or thrombocytopenia.

Available Prepared Suppositories include:

- Morphine [Upsher–Smith] – 5, 10, 20, or 30 mg,
- Hydormorphone (Dilaudid) [Knoll] – 3 mg, and
- Oxymorphone –5 mg.
  (Numorphan) [DuPont Pharmaceuticals]

Transdermal is a new method of administration. It is now on the market in the form of a controlled-release "patch". Duragesic (Janssen) is fentanyl, a short-acting narcotic, which is available as a 72-hour product and clients/families can manage these with ease. There will be a delay of approximately 12 hours until peak level of analgesia is reached and supplemental medications will be required. Transdermal administration may require a trial period to make certain that the dose is correct and that the product does indeed provide analgesia for a 72-hour duration for the client.

The subcutaneous route of administration is often overlooked since caregivers became accustomed to intravenous administration. A small gauge (25 or 27 gauge) butterfly needle can be placed anywhere there is adequate subcutaneous tissue (e.g., abdomen or even thigh if the individual is not ambulatory) and the line may be used continuously or intermittently. The site should be inspected every eight hours for redness, edema and tenderness, but the butterfly needle can be left in place for 5–7 days without changing sites if there are no problems. Ideally, the medication should be concentrated so that there is ≤1 cc infused per hour. It is possible to administer larger amounts if absorption is adequate. Bruera, Legris, Kuehn, and Miller (1990) describe the successful subcutaneous infusion of narcotics and fluids at the rate of 20–100 cc/hr with the addition of hyaluronidase.

Intravenous administration at home may require a permanent central line. Unless the client requires the line for other purposes (e.g., hydration, nutrition, antibiotics), it adds cost without additional benefit over other routes for pain management. If the client cannot swallow, has diarrhea and has inadequate subcutaneous tissue, this may be the route of choice. It can be used intermittently (with a flushing schedule) or continuously via a Patient Controlled Analgesia (PCA) system.

Patient Controlled Analgesia (PCA) is a method of pain control involving a machine-delivery system which is programmed by the nurse and can deliver a basal (continuous) amount with an incremental/bolus (intermittent) amount or a combination of both. This type of technology can be used either subcutaneously or intravenously and allows the patient to have control over this area of life, namely pain management.

The intramuscular route has been used over time for pain management. It is not a route of choice for the person who must receive medications for an extended period of time. Sites may become limited, absorption becomes erratic, and more importantly it requires the added pain of an injection when the intent is to relieve pain.

When a person has been on the other methods of analgesic administration and they are not effective for some reason (e.g., intolerable side effects, high dose levels), a route which may indeed provide relief is via the opiate receptors of the spinal column. The sites may be:

A. Epidural — a catheter is placed between the vertebral column and the dura. The client will require about 1/10 the amount of narcotic as required parenterally.

B. Intrathecal — a catheter is placed between the dura and the arachnoid layers of the meninges. The client will require about 1/100 of the narcotic as required parenterally.

C. Intraventricular — a catheter is placed directly into one of the cerebral ventricles with a reservoir placed under the scalp for refill. The intent is to continuously deliver the medication.

The epidural or intrathecal catheter may be tunneled to the exterior for intermittent injection or a port/pump may be implanted for continuous infusion with a bolus option.

Direct CNS analgesia is a relatively new area in nursing practice. It is wise to determine what your state Nurse Practice Act allows nursing to do regarding an intraspinal catheter (e.g., if nurses may inject, which medications may be injected?) Wilke (1990) advocates the use of preservative-free solutions until research determines whether preservatives are harmful or not. Another area of question is whether to use alcohol or provodone-iodine in cleansing the injection port. Most guidelines state provodone-iodine due to the known toxic effect of alcohol to the spinal cord. (See the American Nurses Association Position Statement on the Role of the Registered Nurse in the Management of Analgesia by Catheter Techniques, American Nurse, February 1992, p. 7).

NONPHARMACOLOGIC INTERVENTIONS

There are activities nurses can teach the client/family which aid in the reduction of pain. Interventions are most effective when the pain level is low. These interventions can be used as an adjunct to medications when the pain is moderate. There is a lack of research to support many of these psychosocial interventions, but they have merit and warrant a trial basis with certain clients.

Nonpharmacologic actions include physical and behavioral interventions. These interventions will be discussed in the following section.

Physical interventions involve cutaneous stimulation, which stimulates the skin for the purpose of relieving pain. These activities include therapeutic touch, pressure, massage, ice, physical therapy, and TENS Units. The nurse plays an important role in teaching these techniques, in assessing whether they are being done correctly and in evaluating whether they are indeed effective.

Behavioral interventions focus the person's mind on something other than the pain sensation. These techniques are individualized to the person's preference. Behavioral interventions will be effective only when the person believes that they will work. Relaxation, distraction, imagery, visualization, music, humor, prayer, education, play therapy (for children), biofeedback, and hypnosis are behavioral interventions.

In order for these interventions to be effective, the nurse must explore the interest areas of the client, determine which may have meaning for the client, and assess the client's belief that the approach will make a difference in relieving pain. Each technique requires time to teach and practice before becoming effective.

Relaxation is a state of relative freedom from both anxiety and skeletal tension. Examples include distracting thoughts, rhythmic breathing, peaceful images, quiet environment and repetition.

Distraction focuses on stimuli other than the pain sensation. This is often done without realizing that it is a form of analgesia and is reducing the sensation of pain. Some examples include music (auditory distraction), tapping (tactile distraction), TV or flowers (visual distraction), people and humor. These activities may be employed with little or no cost and used as an adjunct to medications.

Imagery/visualization use one's imagination. This may focus on a close person, a place of enjoyment, a past event, or anything which is thought to bring pleasure. Examples of imagery are emptying the sandbag, breathing out pain, and a ball of healing energy. The mind is occupied and therefore the pain reduces in focus.

The use of music (tapes, records, CDs, live performances) take the thoughts away from the painful sensation. This is very individual. The person's preference and the client's choice must be explored. A teenager's choice of music would probably not be the choice of the person over 70 and the person trained in classical music may not be a country/western fan.

Humor can provide immediate distraction, but it also can provide prolonged pain relief, even up to two hours. Does the person have a favorite comedian? Are there audio or visual recordings available of that person performing? Is there a joke book which would match the person's sense of humor? Encourage the use of humor as many people who experience an ongoing pain find that they have little about which to laugh.

Prayer uses communication with a higher power. The client's religious beliefs need to be explored. Is the person a Christian and accustomed to talking with God? Is the person a Hindu for whom there are many gods? Is the person a Moslem who prays to Allah? Is the person an atheist for whom there is no god or higher power and for whom this would not be an option?

The use of games or toys is play therapy. This can be useful for children, but also for adults. To play is to involve the person physically and mentally in an activity and thus provide distraction. To a child, dolls can become the object taking on the pain. To an adult, a board game may provide competition and focus.

Biofeedback is the ability to alter the body functions (e.g., heart rate, blood pressure, muscle relaxation) by intentional mental focusing. It requires skill of a professional person who is trained in the technique. The person may have utilized this approach in the past and it is worth exploring as an adjunct during this time of pain.

The use of psychotherapy to alter the affective and sensory component of pain is hypnosis. This requires a professional skilled in teaching hypnosis. Ahles (1987) questions how effective this technique might be for patients with other than mild to moderate pain. More research is required in this area.

CLIENT/FAMILY EDUCATION
Nurses play a major role in the teaching process. It may be spontaneous, informal, or lengthy with resources. Client education should include:

- Cause of pain
- Anticipated outcome (pain relief)

    Is the Client expecting no pain or manageable pain?
- What to report to MD/RN

    Unmanaged side effects

    Uncontrolled pain
- Medication information (schedule, doses, refills and drug interactions)
- Side effects of medications and what to do to prevent or treat them (e.g., patient may be drowsy the first few days of narcotic use, but this effect will pass)

- Information to restructure attitudes and beliefs regarding addiction, medications, etc.
- Plan for follow-up and who to call for emergency assistance
- Client's and provider's responsibilities for pain management plan

EVALUATION

Once assessment, planning and interventions have been implemented, evaluation then proceeds to determine effectiveness of pain management. Ways to evaluate pain vary, important aspects to include in an evaluation include:

- Daily Pain Diary
- Level of Satisfaction with the pain control
- Side Effects

SIDE EFFECT MANAGEMENT

Side effects are expected to be managed effectively. Constipation is a side effect that does not diminish over time. It will require treatment consistently and prophylactically. If there are not orders for a bowel regimen, obtain them.

Assess the following:

1. bowel sounds of good quality
2. an established bowel pattern (at least q 2 days)
3. Some of the products to include in a bowel program are:

> docusate sodium — a stool softener which lowers surface tension, permitting water and fats to penetrate and soften stools.
>
> senna — a natural laxative vegetable derivative from the Cassia plant; induces peristalsis — classed as a mild laxative.
>
> bisacodyl — a contact laxative which stimulates sensory nerves to produce parasympathetic reflexes resulting in increased peristaltic contractions of the colon.
>
> magnesium citrate — a bowel evacuant which prevents the intestine from absorbing water; be aware that this may produce dehydration.
>
> lactulose — a synthetic disaccharide. The metabolites of bacterial action on the lactulose increases water.

Three recommended regimens for persons being treated for cancer pain are:

1. T. Decan Walsh, 1990, offers the SOS plan:

> S — Stool softener (docusate sodium-Colace)
> O — Osmotic laxative (Milk of Magnesia)
> S — Stimulant laxative (bisacodyl - Dulcolax)

2. American Pain Society, 1989, recommends:

    docusate sodium (Colace) 100-300 mg/day + senna (Senokot)

3. The Texas Cancer Plan, 1990 suggests:

    I. Senokot-S 4 tabs BID to TID

    II. Lactulose 30 ml QD or BID

Nausea/Vomiting

In a study conducted by Campora, Merlini & Pace (1991), 18% of patients on morphine had moderate to severe nausea and 28% experienced emesis. Twenty-five percent of all patients will experience nausea and/or vomiting initially. This side effect decreases after 2–3 days as tolerance develops. Treat the side effect aggressively; it may require ATC (around the clock) management for 1–2 weeks. Antiemetic trials are warranted if nausea or vomiting are a problem.

Possible antiemetics include:

hydroxyzine (Vistaril, Atarax)	25–50 mg q4–6h
prochlorperazine (Compazine)	5–20 mg q4–6h
thiethylperazine (Norzine, Torecan)	10 mg q8h
If patient is too sedated, haloperidol (Haldol)	0.5 – 1.0 mg q4–8h
If sedation is desired, chlorpromazine (Thorazine)	10–25 mg q4h
If gastric stasis is contributory, metoclopramide (Reglan)	30–80 mg/day

According to the APS, 1989, hydroxyzine (Vistaril, Atarax) has analgesic, antiemetic and mild sedative activity in addition to its antihistamine effects.

Sedation

Once pain management is achieved, do not confuse normal extended sleep patterns with sedation. The person may be exhausted from interrupted sleep patterns due to previous pain and may in fact sleep for extended periods initially just to 'catch up'. Assess if the person is alert and oriented when awake. Determine if the person has established a good nighttime sleep pattern and the person can be aroused from sleep.

Stimulants can be added to the pain management program if sedation is a problem. See page 144 for examples and dosing.

Confusion and/or hallucinations are most often temporary. Impaired renal function will have an impact on the clearance of the narcotics. Tolerance to these side effects usually develop within 48–72 hours.

The client/family should be comfortable with the level of alertness. If this is troublesome in any way, intervention may be necessary. Brain metastases could be another reason for the confusion and/or hallucination.

Pruritis

This intense itching is more often observed with the administration of intraspinal narcotics. It is not frequently seen with the other routes. The person will exhibit this first on the face and may be unconsciously rubbing or scratching at the nose or cheeks. This can be managed with an antihistamine or with even a dilute infusion of a mixed agonist/antagonist or naloxone. Pruritis is not life-threatening, but is certainly bothersome. Nursing intervention will certainly enhance the comfort level of the client.

Respiratory Depression

Tolerance to this potential side effect develops rapidly. The Texas Cancer Plan (1991) states that we have an inordinate fear of respiratory depression. Pain is a natural antagonist to the respiratory depressant effects of opiates and pain provides a natural stimulant. A sleeping rate of 6–8 respirations per minute may be perfectly normal in the totally relaxed person. The 'arousable factor' is a satisfactory guide: Can you arouse the person from sleep? This will stimulate respirations. "New respiratory symptoms are virtually never a primary drug effect in those receiving stable doses of narcotics" according to Portenoy and Coyle, 1990. When doses are escalated, respirations should be monitored for any drastic change. Remind the family members to do this, but do not frighten them. Respiratory depression due to the use of narcotics in cancer pain management is rare. Assessment questions to ask:

What is the respiratory rate? What is the quality of respirations?

Does the client/family understand that respiratory depression is a rare occurrence with continued use of opioids or are they frightened that they may be promoting death?

PEDIATRIC PAIN ISSUES

The treatment of pediatric cancer pain requires special knowledge and skills. All of the principles covered thus far apply to this population. The nurse must also have the knowledge of pediatric dose calculations. Appendix 7 gives examples of pediatric pain assessment tools.

Cahill, Panzarella & Spross (1990) have written a section on "Pediatric Cancer Pain" in the ONS Position Paper on Cancer Pain.

Table 6.5 outlines the myths held about pediatric pain.

TABLE 6.5

MYTHS OF CHILDREN'S PAIN

1. Childrens' nervous systems are not the same as adults', and therefore, children do not experience pain with the intensity that adults do
2. Active children cannot be in pain
3. It is unsafe to administer narcotics to children because they become addicted
4. Narcotics always depress respirations in children
5. Children always tell you if they have pain
6. Children cannot tell you where they hurt
7. The best way to administer analgesics is by injection
8. Parents know all the answers about childrens' pain
9. The child is crying because he/she is restrained, not because he/she is hurting

Cahill et al (1990) identify the following important factors that nurses employ for successful pain management in the pediatric population. Nursing strategies include:

1. Believe that children, even very young children, experience pain
2. Recognize that children remember painful experiences
3. Include the aid of parents/significant others in comforting/relieving pain and in helping the child cope with pain
4. Incorporate relaxation strategies into care plans for prevention and treatment of pain in children. (these can be used by children as young as 5 years old)
5. Use distraction techniques as adjunct therapy for pediatric pain, not as primary therapy. Children use distraction very effectively, which may lead parents and providers to believe that the child is not in pain or that the pain is not severe. However, do not assume that the success of distraction means that the pain, or the distress associated with it, is gone
6. Always be honest with children and explain procedures truthfully, including information about whether the procedures will hurt.
7. Initiate discussion about pain with children/parents. Remind them that nurses, doctors, and others do not necessarily know when the child has pain

GERIATRIC PAIN ISSUES

A segment of our population which has been often overlooked in the management of pain is the elderly. With the increase in longevity and the resultant 'aging population' we must, as health professionals, develop a more acceptable attitude toward administering pain medications and controlling pain in the elderly.

McCaffrey and Beebe (1989) have a chapter devoted to this topic with explanations and recommendations. Some of the myths which impede health care professionals in adequately managing pain in the elderly are:

1. Pain is a natural outcome of growing old.

2. Pain perception, or sensitivity, decreases with age.

3. The potential side effects of narcotics make them too dangerous to use to relieve pain in the elderly.

4. If the elderly client appears to be occupied, sleeps, or can be otherwise distracted from pain, then he does not have much pain.

5. If the older person is depressed, especially if there is no known cause for the pain, then depression is causing the pain. Pain is a symptom of depression and would subside if the depression were effectively treated.

6. Narcotics are totally inappropriate for all clients with chronic nonmalignant pain.

The nurse should keep in mind the following physiological realities when addressing pain in the elderly.

Firstly, the distribution of drugs pharmacokinetically in the elderly differs from that of younger people. As aging occurs there are changes in the body composition, an increase of fat and decrease in heart, kidney and muscle mass. Usual adult doses may need to be decreased to avoid toxic drug levels in the blood and tissue. Decreased circulating proteins due to serum proteins, malnutrition or chronic diseases potentially result in greater drug effect from higher concentrations of unbound drug, with a greater risk of toxic effect.

Secondly the metabolism of drugs. There is limited research in the area of hepatic metabolic rates in relation to aging. It may be safer to allow for longer intervals between doses in the elderly.

Finally, the excretion of drugs change due to a decrease in renal mass, renal blood flow, glomerular filtration rate, and tubular secretion. All these changes occur in the kidney due to aging. With reduced function, the drugs or their active metabolites may remain in the body longer.

When working with an elderly population, analgesics are appropriate for pain management. Consider decreasing the dosage in this population. The interval between doses may need to be lengthened and the frequency of assessment and evaluation must be increased.

Nursing interventions include accurate assessment, titrate to the effect, and intervene exactly as one would for other age groups.

CONCLUSION

Angarola & Donato (1991) report that a jury awarded $15 million in damages to a family as a result of nursing actions which caused increased pain and suffering through withholding narcotics during terminal illness. Pain management is becoming a quality of care issue.

NOT ONLY CAN YOU MAKE A DIFFERENCE IN SUCCESSFUL CANCER PAIN MANAGEMENT FOR THE CLIENT AT HOME, YOU DO MAKE THE DIFFERENCE.

BIBLIOGRAPHY

Ahles, T. (1987). Psychological techniques for the management of cancer-related pain. In D.B. McGuire & C.H. Yarbro (eds). *Cancer Pain Management.* New York: Grune & Stratton, Inc.

American Hospital Formulary Service. (1991). Opiate Agonists. Bethesda, MD: American Society of Hospital Pharmacists, p 1148.

American Pain Society. (1989). *Principles of analgesic use in the treatment of acute pain and chronic cancer pain — a concise guide to medical practice. 2nd edition.* (Copies available through the American Pain Society, PO Box 186, Skokie, IL 60076-0186).

Angarola, R.T. & Donato, B.J. (1991). Inappropriate pain management results in high jury award. (letter). *Journal of Pain and Symptom Management, 6* (7), 407.

Bruera, E., Brenneis, C., Paterson, A.H. & MacDonald, R.N. (1989). Use of methylphenidate as an adjuvant to narcotic analgesics in patients with advanced cancer. *Journal of Pain and Symptom Management, 4* (1), 3–6.

Bruera, E., Legris, M.A., Kuehn, N. & Miller, M.J. (1990). Hypodermoclysis for the administration of fluids and narcotic analgesics in patients with advanced cancer. *Journal of Pain and Symptom Management, 5* (4), 218-220.

Campora, E., Merlini, L., Pace, M., Bruzzone, M., Luzzani M., Gottlieb, A. & Rosso, R. (1991). The incidence of narcotic-induced emesis. *Journal of Pain and Symptom Management. 6* (7), 428–430.

Cleeland, C., Foley, K.M. & Levy, M.H. (1989) Stepped management of cancer pain. *Patient Care,* February 15, pp 170–186.

Cohen, F.L. Postsurgical pain relief: Patients' status and nurses' medication choices. *Pain, 9,* 265-274.

Cole, L. & Hanning, C.D. (1990). Review of the rectal use of opioids. *Journal of Pain and Symptom Management, 5*(2), 118—126.

Consensus Development Conference of NIH. (1987). The integrated approach to the management of pain. *Journal of Pain and Symptom*

Management, 2 (1), 35–41.

Dalton, J.A. (1989). Nurses' perceptions of their pain assesment skills, pain management practices, and attitudes toward pain. *Oncology Nursing Forum, 16*(2), 225-231.

Donovan, M.I. (1989). An historical view of pain management: how we got to where we are! *Cancer Nursing, 12*(4), 257–261.

Dundee, J.W. & Moore, J. (1961). The myth of phenothiazine potentiation. *Anesthesiology 16,* 95–96.

Enck, R.E. (1990). Parenteral narcotics for pain control in the homecare environment. *Caring 9* (5), 38–41.

Ferrell, B.R. & Schneider, C. (1988). Experience and management of cancer pain at home. *Cancer Nursing, 11*(2), 84–90.

Ferrell, B.R. & Ferrell, B.A. (July/August 1990). Easing the pain. *Geriatric Nursing,* 175—178.

Guidelines for Treatment of Cancer Pain. Final Report of the Texas Cancer Council's Workgroup on Pain Control in Cancer Patients. (1991). Texas Cancer Council.

Inturrisi, C.E. (1984). Pharmacology of narcotic analgesics. *Symposium on the Management of Cancer Pain,* New York: HP Publishing Co., Inc. 22–29.

Inturrisi, C.E. (1989). Management of cancer pain — Pharmacology and principles of management. *Cancer 63* (11), 2308–2320.

Kaiko, R.F., Foley, K.M., Grabinski, P.Y., et al. (1983). Central nervous system excitatory effects of meperidine in cancer patients. *Annals of Neurology, 13,* 180–185.

Kaiko, R.F. (1985). Heroin: Facts and comparisons. *PRN Forum, 4,* 1–2.

Lapin, J., Portenoy, R.K., Coyle, N., Houde, R.W. & Foley, K.M. (1989). Guidelines for use of controlled-release oral morphine in cancer pain management: correlation with clinical experience. *Cancer Nursing, 12* (4), 202–208.

Marks, R. & Sachar, E. (1973). Undertreatment of medical inpatients with narcotic analgesics. *Annals of Internal Medicine, 78,* 173–181.

McCaffery, M. & Beebe, A. (1989). *Pain: A Clinical Manual for Nursing Practice.* St. Louis: C.V. Mosby Company.

McCaffery, M. (1990). Pain management: Nurses lead the way to new priorities. *American Journal of Nursing, 90* (10), 45–49.

McGee, J.L. & Alexander, M.R (May 1979). Phenothiazine analgesia — fact or fantasy? *American Journal of Hospital Pharmacy, 36:* 633–640.

McGuire, D.B. & Yarbro, C.H. (1987). Cancer Pain Management. New

York: Grune & Stratton, Inc.

McGuire, D.B. (1989). Cancer pain: Pathophysiology of pain in cancer. *Cancer Nursing, 12*(5), 310–315.

McLaughlin-Hagan, M. (1990). Continuous subcutaneous infusion of narcotics. *Journal of Intravenous Nursing, 13* (2), 119-121.

Paice, J.A. (1988). The phenomenon of analgesic tolerance in cancer pain management. *Oncology Nursing Forum, 15* (4), 455–460.

Paice, J.A. (1991). Unraveling the mystery of pain. *Oncology Nursing Forum, 18* (5), 843–849.

Porter, J. & Jick, H. (1980). Addiction rate in patients treated with narcotics (letter). *New England Journal of Medicine,* 302: 123.

Portenoy, R.K. & Coyle, N. (1990). Controversies in the long-term management of analgesic therapy in patients with advanced cancer. *Journal of Pain and Symptom Management, 5*(5), 307–319.

Portenoy, R.K. (1989). Cancer pain — Epidemiology & syndromes. *Cancer 63* (11), 2298–2307.

Relieving Pain: An analgesic guide. Principles of analgesic use in the treatment of acute pain and chronic cancer pain. American Cancer Society. (1988). *American Journal of Nursing, 88* (6), 815–825.

Rogers, A.G. (1990). The successful use of controlled-release morphine. *Journal of Pain and Symptom Management, 5*(5), 331–332.

Spross, J.A., McGuire, D.B. & Schmitt, R.M. (1990). Oncology Nursing Society Position Paper on Cancer Pain — Part I (Scope of Nursing Practice Regarding Cancer Pain, Ethics and Practice). *Oncology Nursing Forum, 17* (4), 595–614.

Spross, J.A., McGuire, D.B. & Schmitt, R.N. (1990). Oncology Nursing Society Position Paper on Cancer Pain — Part II (Education, Research and list of cancer pain management resources). *Oncology Nursing Forum, 17* (5), 751–760.

Spross, J.A., McGuire, D.B. & Schmitt, R.N. (1990). Oncology Nursing Society Position Paper on Cancer Pain — Part III (Nursing Administration, Pediatric Cancer Pain and Appendices). *Oncology Nursing Forum, 17* (6), 943–955.

Swenson, C.J., Sikorski, K., DeWaters, T. + Bucknell Ryan, S. (1991). Narcotic oral equivalents. *Oncology Nursing Forum, 18*(5), 942.

Thorpe, D.M. (1990). Comprehensive pain care: The relief of pain and suffering. *Dimensions in Oncology Nursing, 4* (1), 27–29.

Twycross, R.G. & Lack, S.A. (1990). *Oral morphine: Information for Patients, Friends and Families.* Beaconsfield, Bucks, England: Beaconsfield Publishers, Ltd. (Available through Roxane Laboratories, Inc.)

Walsh, T.D. (1990). Prevention of opioid side effects. *Journal of Pain and*

Symptom Management, 5 (6), 362–367.

Watt-Watson, J.H. (1987). Nurses' knowledge of pain issues: A survey. *Journal of Pain and Symptom Management, 2,* 207–211.

Weissman, D.E., Burchman, S.L., Dinndorf, P.A. & Dahl, J.L. (1990). Handbook of Cancer Pain Management (2nd edition). From the Medical College of Wisconsin and the University of Wisconsin Medical School in conjunction with The Wisconsin Pain Initiative.

Wilke, D.J. (1990). Cancer pain management: State-of-the-art nursing care. *Nursing Clinics of North America, 25* (2), 331–343.

Vascular Access Devices

Suzanne F. Herbst, RN, MA
NMC Homecare, Syracuse, N.Y.

VASCULAR ACCESS DEVICES

Suzanne F. Herbst, RN, MA
NMC Homecare, Syracuse, N.Y.

INTRODUCTION

Since the first clinical use of intravenous chemotherapy and the continuous development of sophisticated pharmaceuticals, venous access has become the mainstay for treatment and supportive care for many persons with cancer. The greatest challenge for the oncology nurse is to maintain adequate access in a patient population that requires frequent therapies and blood sampling. Multiple venipunctures put patients at risk for infection, peripheral vein damage, or extravasation; subject patients to painful searches for a vein; induce fear of injections; and place stress on the nurse.

As a result of the technical revolution, a plethora of vascular access devices are available as alternatives to multiple painful venipunctures. Choices range from small gauge (20 -26 ga.) percutaneously inserted single lumen catheters to large gauge (10-13 ga.) surgically implanted multilumen devices.

In 1991 it was estimated that the vascular access device (VAD) market exceeded 300 million dollars in sales. Made by over 30 manufacturers, each VAD has its own unique characteristics and features. Staying abreast of evolving technology requires multidisciplinary communication in order to share experiences and enhance the care of patients with VAD's. Ironically, although many health care providers are barely comfortable using VAD's, their use and maintenance is already being turned over to patients and nonprofessional caregivers. Oncology nurses play a vital role in patient and caregiver education.

CLASSIFICATION AND DESCRIPTION OF DEVICES

When venous access is ordered or discussed, a variety of terminologies are used inconsistently, creating a great deal of confusion. This section will identify device classifications and descriptions in order to facilitate understanding between author and user.

Vascular Access Devices (VAD's) provide venous access for blood sampling and for administration of fluids, drugs and blood products. VAD's are divided into three major classifications:

- Non-Tunneled Catheters
- Tunneled Catheters
- Implanted Ports

These three major types of VAD's are illustrated in Figure 7.1.

Figure 7.1

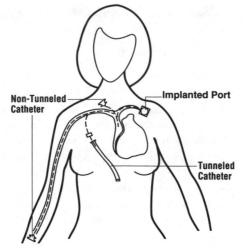

Non-Tunneled Catheter

Implanted Port

Tunneled Catheter

Drawn by Philip J. Quinn

NON-TUNNELED CATHETERS

Non-tunneled catheters are inserted percutaneously via the central venous system of the neck and chest, or via the peripheral venous system of the hand, arm, or foot. Non-tunneled catheters are known as central venous access catheters or peripheral venous access catheters.

Central Venous Access Catheters

This type of catheter has been used traditionally in critical care as a central venous pressure (CVP) line. They are often referred to as "CVP lines" or "Subclavian catheters". Insertion sites of choice for these catheters are:

- High internal jugular
- External jugular
- Low internal jugular
- Supraclavicular
- Infraclavicular

These catheters are usually sutured in place, and if made of silicone or polyurethane, are best suited for short term use (two to three months). This type of catheter may be safely used for immunosuppressed patients that would not be able to tolerate a surgical procedure to insert another type of device.

These types of catheters are available in single, double or triple lumens. The advantages and disadvantages of central venous access catheters are highlighted in Table 7.1.

Peripheral Venous Access

Short Term Peripheral IV Cannulae

Although most persons requiring extensive infusion therapy have a long term vascular access device in place, short term peripheral cannulae are still used in significant numbers. In a recent nationwide survey, Dibble and Ryder report that 79% of adults and 63% of children hospitalized had a peripheral IV, whereas, 19% of adults and 10% of children treated at home had a peripheral IV.

TABLE 7.1

Advantages / Disadvantages of Central Venous Access Catheters

Advantages

- Surgical procedure with patient sedation not required
- Insertion site easily covered with clothing
- Catheter may be exchanged over a guide wire if catheter is damaged or sepsis related to catheter is suspected
- Easily removed at completion of therapy

Disadvantages

- Insertion technique puts patients at risk for: pneumothorax, hemothorax, hydrothorax, arterial puncture, tracheal injury, thoracic duct injury, nerve plexus damage, catheter migration, myocardial perforation and death
- Sterile dressing technique used requiring higher skill level for maintenance care and increased cost of supplies
- Swimming not permitted
- Suture sites may become irritated

The most commonly used short term device is the over-the-needle catheter which is left in place 48-72 hours or until removal is necessary. Insertion requires venipuncture and threading of the catheter over the needle into the vein, removing the needle and leaving just the catheter in place. Steel cannulae or Butterflies® are rarely used for continuous infusions, but are an excellent choice for short bolus infusions or blood sampling.

Extended Peripheral Catheters

A new polymer called Aquavene®, an elastomeric hydrogel, has allowed for increased dwell time of catheters in peripheral vessels. Outside the body, Aquavene is stiff enough to provide an over-the-needle insertion of the catheter. Once in the vessel this material softens, dramatically reducing the incidence of mechanical phlebitis and infiltration. The inner diameter of this catheter also swells two gauge sizes enhancing greater flow potential. For example, after insertion of a 24 gauge Aquavene® catheter the inner diameter swells to a 22 gauge size.

Midline Catheters

Another type of Aquavene® catheter that has revolutionized peripheral access is the Landmark® Midline Venous Access Device. This over-the-needle catheter may be inserted through the veins of the antecubital space and advanced 2 to 6 inches into the veins in the upper arm. Because the veins in the upper arm are larger than those of the hand and forearm, greater dilution occurs significantly reducing the incidence of irritation and phlebitis. This is an excellent choice for therapies requiring 4 to 6 weeks of infusion. It decreases the number of restarts often necessary with catheters used in the hand and forearms.

Peripherally Inserted Central Catheters (PICC)
The use of PICC lines was introduced in the critical care areas in the 1960's but abandoned because of a high incidence of complications, primarily phlebitis, infection and vessel perforation. With technological improvements in catheter materials and methods of insertion, these types of catheters have gained considerable popularity.

Made of a flexible, soft material such as silicone, polyurethane or other polymer, the PICC line is inserted into a peripheral vein at the antecubital space and threaded into the venous system. Depending on the therapy, the tip may terminate in the superior vena cava or at any predetermined point along the venous system. Catheter designs and placement techniques include the following insertion methods:

- over-the-needle
- break-away-needle
- introducer sheath
- peel-away sheath
- seldinger / modified seldinger

TABLE 7.2

Advantages and Disadvantages of Peripheral Venous Catheters

Advantages

- May be inserted by a nurse
- Eliminates potential complication risks of neck and chest insertions
- More economical as it can be inserted without patient sedation or additional surgery
- PICC lines may be exchanged using a guidewire procedure if catheter needs to be replaced
- Easy removal at completion of therapy

Disadvantages

- Location of catheter limits patients mobility
- No swimming permitted
- Requires sterile dressing procedures
- Patient will need assistance with maintenance procedures
- Daily heparin flushes with most brands

The greatest advantage of the PICC line is that central venous access may be achieved without surgical invasive techniques or risks involved from central placement in the neck and chest.

Most State Board of Registered Nurses permit nurses to insert PICC lines if they have had appropriate education and training. PICC lines may be inserted in a variety of settings including the hospital physician's office, clinic or at home.

Figures 7.2 and 7.3 illustrate the veins of the arm, as well as the anthropometric measurements of the veins as they move centrally to the vena cava.

Figure 7.2

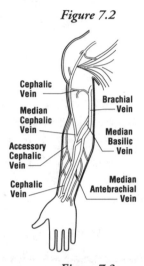

Cephalic Vein

Brachial Vein

Median Cephalic Vein

Median Basilic Vein

Accessory Cephalic Vein

Cephalic Vein

Median Antebrachial Vein

Figure 7.3

VEIN	PROXIMAL DIAMETER	LENGTH
Cephalic	6 mm	38 cm
Basilic	8 mm	24 cm
Axillary	16 mm	13 cm
Subclavian	19 mm	6 cm
R Innominate	19 mm	2.5 cm
L Innominate	19 mm	6 cm
SVC	20 mm	7 cm

TUNNELED CATHETERS

Tunneled catheters were introduced by Dr. Broviac in 1969 followed shortly by the Hickman® catheter. These radiopaque silicone rubber catheters are characterized by a cuff attached to the catheter. These catheters are tunneled into the subcutaneous tissue. In about 7 to 10 days the cuff, made of dacron, and the subcutaneous tissue begin to adhere together creating a secure anchor for the catheter and a mechanical barrier against ascending infection. Historically, these catheters have been called 'right atrial catheters', because the tip was placed in the right atrium of the heart. Recently the Food and Drug Administration Central Venous Catheter-Working Group, in response to an increased incidence of cardiac perforation and tamponade, recommends the lower 1/3 of the superior vena cava as the site for optimal tip placement.

Recently, a new type of cuff called the Vitacuff® is being attached to these catheters in conjunction with the dacron cuff. This leaves 2 cuffs in the subcutaneous tunnel with the Vitacuff® closest to the exit site. The Vitacuff® is a silver impregnated collagen cuff that acts as an antimicrobial for approximately 30 days. Data has shown that the presence of the Vitacuff® has decreased the number of catheter infections related to insertion techniques.

The newest tunneled catheter is the Groshong®, made of thin-walled, translucent silicone with a radiopaque strip and a three-way valve along the side of the distal end. This valve remains closed when not in use and allows for easy infusion or withdrawal. This valve minimizes the potential for air embolism, reduces the risk of blood backflow and requires that the catheter be flushed once a week with saline when not in use.

Tunneled catheters are available in single, double or triple lumens; the advantages and disadvantages of tunneled catheters are listed in Table 7.3.

TABLE 7.3

Advantages / Disadvantages of Tunneled Catheters

Advantages

- Subcutaneous tunnel secures placement of catheter
- Dacron cuff minimizes risk of infection
- External access facilitates use for patient and caregiver without discomfort
- Easily repaired if catheter damaged distal to exit site
- Swimming and bathing allowed after tunnel is well healed, with special instructions

Disadvantages

- Requires invasive surgical insertion
- External portion of catheter visible outside chest
- Requires clean or sterile dressing changes
- Daily heparin flushes necessary except for Groshong® catheters that require weekly saline flushes
- May require simple surgery to remove

IMPLANTED PORTS

Implanted ports consist of a self-sealing dense silicone septum in a titanium, stainless steel or plastic housing and a catheter made of silicone or polyurethane. The silicone septum and housing are surgically implanted in a pocket made in the subcutaneous tissue of the chest and the catheter is threaded into the superior vena cava. Access to the venous system is achieved by aseptically inserting a non-coring needle through the skin and silicone septum into the fluid path.

Another device available is the PAS-PORT®, which is a combination of a peripherally inserted catheter and implanted port. A catheter is percutaneously inserted via the antecubital space and advanced centrally. Catheter placement is facilitated by the use of a catheter tracking device called the Cath-Finder®. The distal end of the catheter is attached to a small, low profile port which is implanted in the antecubital area. Use and maintenance of the PAS-PORT® is very similar to that of the chest implanted ports.

A new port under development called the Cath-Link System™ may be accessed by an angiocatheter instead of a needle. Angiocatheters are more readily available in most health care settings than non-coring needles and are more cost effective. The Cath-Link System may be implanted in the upper arm, utilizing the brachial vein for access or in the standard chest wall location.

Because implanted ports are accessed only when needed, a port is an ideal choice for patients requiring cyclical therapies, such as chemo-therapy. When the port is not in continuous use, it needs to be flushed monthly to maintain patency. Furthermore, many patients prefer ports because its presence is easier to conceal, especially when it is not accessed.

Implanted ports are manufactured with top and side entry access and with single and double lumen systems. Table 7.4 covers the advantages and disadvantages of implanted ports.

DEVICE SELECTION

Oncology nurses are key advocates for patients and caregivers in facilitat-ing the selection of an appropriate vascular access device (VAD). Encour-aging placement of a VAD early in treatment is important. The insertion procedure is better tolerated when a patient's venous system has not been traumatized by previous therapies.

TABLE 7.4

Advantages / Disadvantages of Implanted Ports

Advantages

- System enclosed completely under skin requiring minimal or no care except during continuous infusions
- Requires flushing once a month when not in use
- Increased patient mobility and freedom
- Swimming permitted when not accessed

Disadvantages

- Requires surgical procedure for insertion and removal, increasing costs
- Special non-coring needle required for access
- Discomfort from needle stick when port is accessed
- Difficult and awkward to self-access

Assisting the patient and caregiver in selecting a device requires thoughtful planning and consideration of the following:

- Patient preference
- Physical status of patient
  - visual acuity
  - manual dexterity
  - level of fatigue and weakness
- Psychological status of patient and support persons
- Frequency of access and duration of therapy
- Intellectual ability of patient or caregiver
- Home environment and family support
- Assistance required and available

The following Table 7.5 by Goodman and Wickham will assist the clinicians in prioritizing the need for a VAD.

TABLE 7.5

Patient Assessment Criteria for a VAD

Criteria

Frequency of Venous Access
Longevity of Treatment
Mode of Administration
Venous Integrity Patient Preference

Low Priority	High Priority
• Infrequent venous access	• Frequent venous access
• Short-term therapy	• Long-term indefinite treatment period
• Intermittent single injections	• Continuous infusion chemotherapy
• Non-vesicant /non-irritating drugs	• Home infusion of chemotherapy
• No previous IV therapy	• Vesicant/irritating drugs
• Both extremities available	• Venous thrombosis/ sclerosis due to previous IV therapy
• Venous access with 2 or fewer venipunctures	• Venous access limited to one extremity
• Patient does not prefer VAD	• Prior tissue damage due to extravasation
	• Multiple (>2) venipunctures to secure venous access Patient prefers VAD

Source: Goodman, Michelle S., Venous Access Devices: An Overview. Oncology Nursing Forum 11(5): 17, 1984. Reprinted with permission from the Oncology Nursing Press. Inc.

TABLE 7.6

Maintenance Summary of Vascular Access Devices

Classification

Tunneled Catheters
Hickman/Broviac
    Heparin strength used?
    Amount of Heparin flush?
    Frequency of irrigation?
    Cap change frequency
    Dressing used
    Frequency of drsg.* change
    Clamping when not in use

Groshong
    No Heparin flush required
    Normal saline flush 5 ml
    Frequency of irrigation,
    Cap change frequency
    Dressing used
    Frequency of drsg.* change
    Clamping when not in use

Implanted Ports
    Heparin strength used
    Amount of Heparin flush?
    Frequency of irrigation?
    when not in use
    No dressing necessary when not in use
    Non coring needle insertion
    Frequency of needle change (continuous infusion)

Non-tunneled Catheters
    Heparin strength used
    Amount of Heparin flush?
    Frequency of irrigation?
    Cap change frequency
    Dressing used
    Frequency of drsg. * change

* Depends on dressing used.
Reference: Herbst, S. Care of the HIV Patient with a Vascular Access Device, In: Lewis, Angie (Ed) Nursing Care of the Patient with AIDS/ARC, Aspen, 1988.

Summary of Nursing Surveys: S.F. Bay Area Vascular Access Network
Oncology Nursing Society - 1987 Congress Vascular Access Device
Workshop

Most Popular	to	Least
100 u/ml	10 u/ml	1000 u/ml
3 ml or >	2.5 ml	< 2.5 ml
QD	BID	QOD
weekly		as needed
occlusive	gauze/tape	none
weekly	QOD	daily
never		always
weekly and after each use		
weekly		as needed
occlusive	gauze/tape	none
weekly	QOD	daily
never		
100 u/ml	1000 u/ml	10u/ml
5 ml	< 5 ml	> 5 ml
after each use		
monthly	> 1 month	weekly
with sterile gloves		no gloves
weekly	<1 week	> 1 week
	5 days	up to 30 days
100 u/ml		
1 ml	2 ml	> 2.5 ml
QD	BID	QOD
weekly		as needed
Occlusive	gauze/tape	none
weekly	QOD	daily

MAINTENANCE

Maintenance procedures are similar for all VAD's. Non-tunneled catheters and implanted ports are cared for according to sterile technique, while clean technique suffices for tunneled catheters after 7 to 10 days when tunnel is well healed. In order to determine the safety and efficacy of maintenance procedures it is imperative to have a quality assurance program in place that looks at problems encountered and complication rates.

The summary of maintenance procedures (Table 7.6) demonstrates the controversies and lack of standardizations within these procedures.

COMPLICATION MANAGEMENT

Vascular Access Devices play a paramount role in the treatment and supportive care of the oncology patient. Despite superior designs and meticulous care, complications still exist in this high risk patient population.

Insertion techniques for centrally placed VAD's put patients at risk for the following complications:

- Pneumothorax
- Subclavian artery injury
- Air embolism
- Catheter embolism
- Venous thrombosis
- Catheter tip misplacement
- Brachial plexus injury
- Hydrothorax
- Thoracic duct laceration
- Hemothorax
- Carotid artery injury

The following are the most frequently reported post - insertion complications:

- Catheter Migration
- Venous Thrombosis
- Catheter Occlusions
- Infection - local or systemic

One of the first clinical manifestations of catheter migration, venous thrombosis, and catheter occlusions is the inability to withdraw blood and/ or inability to infuse. (Refer to Complication Management/Troubleshooting Guide in Appendix 8.)

Other reported complications include:

- Extravasation
- Damaged Catheter
- Air embolism

Catheter Migration/Malposition

Despite optimal catheter tip placement in the superior vena cava, verified by x-ray, catheters migrate or become malpositioned during insertion and use.

Lum (1989) reports that the incidence of malposition or migration of catheter tips vary from 5.5 - 29% via the subclavian vein approach and increase to 21 - 55% via the antecubital vein approach. Factors influencing the incidence of malposition are any increase or change in intrathoracic pressure from coughing, sneezing or vomiting.

Often malpositioned catheters are needlessly removed when safe and effective repositioning techniques are available. If attempts at repositioning fail and the catheter continues to malfunction, removal of catheter may be necessary.

Venous Thrombosis

The biocompatability of catheter materials has been greatly improved—with less thrombogenic properties. The presence of a catheter in the vein still creates a foreign body response. This response is characterized by inflammation of the vessel wall and forming of a fibrin sheath around the catheter. Lindblad (1988) reports that fibrin sleeve formation existed in 66 to 100% of patients studied. The presence of the fibrin sheath promotes the continued deposit of platelets resulting in venous thromobosis or thrombophlebitis. This phenomena presents as phlebitis in peripheral vessels and is apparent and treatable. Central vein thrombophlebitis is subclinical with an incidence reported by Bothe (1991) as high as 68% in patients studied.

Treatment interventions for catheter related venous thrombosis depend on the clinical status and overall patient condition. Clinical interventions include the following:

- Anticoagulation therapy with heparin
- Low dose warfarin
- Fibrinolytic therapy *
- Removal of device

* This approach tends to be less successful if clot has been present for a long time.

Catheter Occlusions

Most catheter occlusions are caused by the following:

- "Pinch off" syndrome
- Intracatheter clot
- Intracatheter precipitate

"Pinch off" Syndrome

This syndrome is primarily associated with catheters that are inserted between the clavicle and first rib. After insertion, as the patient changes positions, the catheters may become pinched or compressed by the changes in the angle between the clavicle and first rib. The danger of this is that the catheter could eventually be fractured resulting in a catheter embolism.

Intracatheter Clot

Intracatheter clot or thrombus formation may develop spontaneously or gradually over time. Prior to the introduction of thrombolytic agents, occluded catheters had to be removed. Most intracatheter clots respond to the local instillation of urokinase 5,000 iu/ml. Urokinase is a protein enzyme produced by the kidney and found in the urine. Before the use of urokinase, streptokinase was used with several adverse reactions being reported. To date, no adverse reactions with urokinase have been reported.

Lawson (1982) reports a 98.6% success rate of declotting catheters after one or two instillations of urokinase 5,000 iu/ml (1 -2 mls), leaving the urokinase in the catheter for 15-30 minutes.

A recent study presented by Fraschini (1991) demonstrates that the use of urokinase instead of the traditional heparin lock devices has dramatically decreased the incidence of catheter occlusions and infection. This promising data is undergoing further investigation.

Intracatheter Precipitate

Often if catheter occlusions do not respond to thrombolytic therapy it may be due to incompatible drug and fluid precipitates. These precipitates or crystalline deposits may respond to the instillation of 1-2ml of the following:

Precipitate	Solution to Instill
• Mineral Precipitate (low ph) (Testerman, 1991)	• Hydrochloric Acid (0.1 N HCL)
• Medication Precipitate (high ph) (Goodwin, 1991)	• Sodium Bicarbonate (1 mEq./ml)
• Lipid Precipitate	• Ethyl Alcohol 70%

Infection

Incidence of catheter related infection rates have been reported in the literature from 2 - 27% (Henderson, 1988). It is difficult to quantitate this information because each author tends to use a different definition of catheter related sepsis (CRS). The following summary by Merritt indicates the range of criteria used to diagnose CRS.

Criteria for the Diagnosis of Catheter-Related Sepsis

Definitive Criteria

1. Positive blood culture (≥ 2) from the catheter and peripheral sites with the same organism isolated from the catheter tip on removal.

2. Persistently positive blood cultures from the catheter and negative cultures from peripheral sites associated with clinical signs of sepsis.

3. Quantitative blood cultures simultaneously collected from the catheter and peripheral sites which show a concentration of organisms 5-10 times as great in the catheter sample as compared to the peripheral sample.

4. Infection at the exit site or tunnel wound due to the same organism as isolated from the blood culture.

Probable Criteria

1. Positive blood cultures from the catheter and/or peripheral sites associated with clinical signs of sepsis which resolve after removal of the line. No other sites of infection are apparent.

2. Positive blood cultures from the catheter and/or peripheral sites associated with a thrombus on the catheter tip. No other source of infection is apparent.

3. Persistently positive blood cultures from the catheter and/or peripheral sites associated with clinical signs of sepsis. No other source of infection is apparent.

Possible Criteria

1. A single positive blood culture from the catheter or peripheral site associated with clinical signs of sepsis without another source of infection apparent.

2. Clinical signs of sepsis without an obvious source which resolve on catheter removal.

Source: Merritt, Nutrition, Vol. 4, No. 3, May/June 1988, p. 247. Reprinted with permission.

The following factors developed by Maki have become the "gold standard" in differentiating CRS from other septic syndromes:

Factors Differentiating Catheter-Associated Bacteremia from other Septic Syndromes*

- Signs and/or symptoms of inflammation at catheter insertion site

- Lack of another source for bacteremia

- Bacteremia occurring in patient otherwise at no risk

- Localized embolic disease distal to arterial catheter

- Hematogenous *Candida* endophthalmitis or other focal *Candida* infections in patients receiving TPN

- Presence of 15 or more colonies of bacteria on semiquantitative culture of catheter tip

- Sepsis apparently refractory to appropriate antimicrobial therapy

- Resolution of signs and symptoms immediately following removal of catheter

- Microbial clues: e.g., typical for catheter-acquired infection (S. aureus, coagulase-negative staphylococci), or typical for infusion or environmental reservoir

- Clustered infection caused by infusion-related organism

*Modified from Maki DG, Goldman DA, Rhame FA: Infection Control in Intravenous Therapy, Ann Intern Med, 79: 867-887, 1973. Reprinted with permission.

The following diagram illustrates the common sites of origin for CRS.

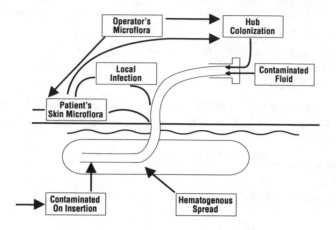

Sites of origin of Vascular Access Devices Infections

Common organisms associated with CRS are:

coagulase-negative staphylococci
staphylococcus aureus
streptococcus species
Klebsiella species
Escherichia coli
Candida species

Risk Factors Influencing CRS include:

Patient Characteristics
- Age
- Severity of disease process
- Degree of immunosuppression
- Presence of other infections

Therapy
- Characteristics of infusates
- Number of drugs
- Frequency and duration of therapy

Catheter Properties
- Size of catheter diameter
- Type and site of insertion
- Number of lumens
- Catheter materials
- Catheter function

Maintenance
- Skin prep/cleansing
- Dressing materials
- Length of needle dwell
- Frequency of access
- Use of in-line filters
- Junction care
- Treatment

The following chart indicates empiric treatment for CRS.

Empiric Antimicrobial Treatment of Central Venous Catheter Sepsis

	Possible Organism	Antibiotic of Choice	Alternative
Community Acquired Infection	Staph aureus S. epidermidis Strep species Gram Negative	Nafcillin + Aminoglycoside	Vancomycin + Aminoglycoside or 3rd generation Cephalosporin
Nosocomial Infections	NSRA NRSE Gram Negative	Vancomycin + Aminoglycoside	Vancomycin + 3rd generation Cephalosporin
Immunocompromised	Gram Positive Gram Negative Pseudomonas	Vancomycin + Extended Spectrum Penicillin + Aminoglycoside	Vancomycin + Ceftazidime +/- Aminoglycoside or Imipenem + Aminoglycoside
Fungal Infection	Candida	Amphotericin B	?

Source: Alvin F. Wong, PharmD, UCSF, Division of Clinical Pharmacy. Reprinted with Permission.

Extravasation

Extravasation is the leakage of a vesicant or irritant drug into the subcutaneous tissue that is capable of causing pain, necrosis, and/or sloughing of tissue.

Although VAD's are often inserted to prevent extravasations, they still occur in small numbers. Whenever a peripheral vein of the hand or arm is used to infuse a vesicant or irritant it is important to select a vein distally and move proximally. Leakage of drug resulting in extravasation may occur if an unsuccessful venipuncture has been performed proximal to the successful venipuncture.

When using a VAD to infuse vesicants or irritants, it is imperative to achieve a blood return prior to infusing the drug. If blood return is not achieved, troubleshooting to determine proper placement and functioning of device must be done prior to initiating infusion.

Extravasations may be caused by:

- a displaced non-coring needle from a port
- separation of catheter from implanted port
- damaged catheter in tunnel area
- fibrin sleeve along catheter allowing back tracking of drug

Prior to the administration of any vesicant or irritant a protocol for treating an extravasation must be reviewed.

The following is a list of vesicant and irritant chemotherapeutic agents. (ONS Cancer Chemotherapy Guideline, 1988).

Vesicants	Irritants
Actinomycin D	BCNU
Cerubidine	DTIC
Adriamycin	VP-16-213/ VePesid
Mutamycin	Zanosar
Estracyte	VM-26
Nitrogen Mustard	Methyl-GAG
Velban	
Oncovin	

Damaged Catheter

When a catheter becomes separated or damaged with an implanted port, the entire system must be removed and replaced. If a non-tunneled catheter is damaged it may be replaced by an over-the-guide wire exchange. If the external portion of a tunneled catheter (single or multi-lumen) is damaged, a repair may be achieved utilizing the appropriate repair kit supplied by the manufacturer. The most important issue is to know the size and type of catheter that needs to be repaired.

Air Embolism

There is potential for air embolism whenever there is an opening into the venous system. Cyclical negative pressure in the thoracic cavity during respiration facilitates the entry of air into the system. Improved VAD designs and the use of Luer-loks® for all connections has greatly reduced the incidence of this complication. Extreme caution must be taken when entering or "de-accessing" the system.

Symptoms of air embolism include:
- chest pain
- dyspnea
- hypotension
- hypoxia
- cyanosis
- tachycarida
- confusion
- loss of consciousness

If air embolism is suspected, place patient on left side in Trendelenburg position or with legs elevated. Administer oxygen if possible and notify physician.

SUMMARY

The manufacturing and use of VAD's continues to increase dramatically. Becoming and staying proficient in the use and maintenance of these devices is extremely challenging but a crucial part of oncology nursing practice. With the multitude of VAD's available, it is imperative that health care professionals communicate and collaborate to achieve optimal outcomes with these devices.

REFERENCES

Askew, A. et al. (1990). Improvement in catheter sepsis rate in burned children. *J Ped Surg, 25(1):117-119.*

Atkinson, J. B., Bagnell, H. A., & Gomperts, E. (1990). Investigational use of tissue plasminogen activator (t-PA) for occluded central venous catheters, *JPEN, 14:*310-311.

Aufweber, E. et al. (1991). Routine semiquantitative cultures and central venous catheter-related bacteremia. *APMIS, 99(*7):627-630.

Babycos, C. et al. (1991). Collodion as a safe, cost-effective dressing for central venous catheters. *S Med J. 83(*11):1286-1287.

Bagnall-Reeb, H.A. & Ruccione, K. (1990). Management of cutaneous reactions and mechanical complications of central venous access devices in pediatric patients with cancer: Algorithms for decision making. *ONF, 17(*5):677-681.

Bailey, E. M., Constance, T. D., Albrecht, L. M. et al. (1990). Coagulase-negative staphylococci: Incidence, pathogenicity, and treatment in the 1990s. *Drug Intell Clin Pharm, 24:*714-720.

Bothe, A. (1991) Catheter-Telated Thrombosis, *Proceedings of 5th Annual NAVAN Conference.*

Bozzetti, F. et al. (1990). Catheter sepsis from infusate contamination. *Nutr Clin Pract, 5*: 156-159.

Brown-Smith, J. K., Stoner, M. H., Barley, Z. A., et al (1990). Tunneled catheter thrombosis: Factors related to incidence. *ONF, 17*(4): 543-549.

Brown, L. H., Wantroba, I., & Simonson, G. (1989). Reestablishing patency in an occluded central venous access device. *Crit Care Nurse, 9*:114-21.

Cahill, S. L. & Benotti, P. N. (1991). Catheter infection control in parenteral nutrition. *Nutr Clin Pract, 6*(2):65-67.

Clarke, D. E. & Raffin, T. A. (1990). Infectious complications of indwelling long-term central venous catheters. *Chest, 97* (4):966-972.

Clifton, G. D. et al. (1991). Comparison of normal saline and heparin solutions for maintenance of arterial patency. *Heart Lung, 20*(2):115-118.

Collignon, P. J. & Munro, R.(1989). Laboratory diagnosis of intravascular catheter associated sepsis. *Eur J.Clin Microbiolol, 8*(9):807-814.

Collins, J. L. et al (1991). In vitro study of simultaneous infusion of incompatible drugs in multilumen catheters. *Heart Lung, 20*(3):271-277.

Corona, M. L. etal. (1990). Infections related to central venous catheters. *Mayo Clin Proc, 65*: 979-986.

Curtas, S. & Tramposch, K. (1991). Culture methods to evaluate central venous catheter sepsis. *Nutr Clin Prac, 6*(2):43-48.

Dawson, S. et al (1991). Right atrial catheters in children with cancer: a decade of experience in the use of tunneled, exteriorized devices at a single institution. *Am J Pediatr Hematol Oncol, 13*(2):126-129.

Dibble, S. and Ryder M. (1991) NAVAN IV study update, *JVAN,* 1(2):9-10.

Duffy, L. F., Kerzner, B., Gebus, V., et al.(1989). Treatment of central venous catheter occlusions with hydrochloric acid. *J Pediatr, 114*: 1002-1004.

Eyer, S. et al. (1990). Catheter-related sepsis: Prospective, randomized study of three methods of long-term catheter maintenance. *Critical Care Med, 18*(10):1073-1079.

Fraschini, G. (1991) Urokinase prophylaxis of central venous ports reduces infectious and thrombotic conplications, *Proceedings of 5th Annual NAVAN Conference.*

Gaillare, J., Merline, R.,Pajot, N. et al. (1990). Conventional and non-conventional modes of vancomycin administration to decontaminate the internal surface of catheters colonized with coagulase-negative staphylococci. *JPEN, 14*:195-200.

Geidel, R. et al. (1991). The percutaneous central venous catheter for small or ill infants. *MCN, 16*:92-96.

Gleason-Morgan, D., et al. (1991). Complications of central venous catheters in pediatric patients with acquired immunodeficiency syndrome. *Ped Infec Dis J, 10*(1):11-14.

Goodwin, M. (119) Using sodium bicarbonate to clear medication precipitate from central venous catheter, *JVAN* 1(2):23.

Goodwin, M. L. (1991). Using sodium bicarbonate to clear a medication precipitate from a central venous catheter. *IVAN*, 1(1):23.

Hadaway, L. (1990). An overview of vascular access devices inserted in the antecubital area. *JIN*, 13(5):297-306.

Haire, W. D. et al. (1990). Obstructed central venous catheters. Restoring function with a 12-hour infusion of low-dose urokinase. *Cancer, Dec.* 1;66(11):2279-2285(39 ref.).

Henderson, D. (1988) Intravascular device - associated infection: current concept and controversies *Infections in Surgery*, 365-399.

Henderson, D. K. (1991). Of snakes and bugs: Nosocomial infection associated with nutritional support. *Nutr Clin Pract*, 6(2):39-41.

Hilton, E. et al.(1988). Central catheter infections: Single-versus triple-lumen catheters. *Am J Med*, 84:667-672.

Horowitz, H.W. et al (1990). Central catheter-related infections: comparison of pulmonary artery catheters and triple lumen catheters for the delivery of hyperalimentation in a critical care setting. *JPEN*, 14(6): 588-592.

Ingram, J., et al. (1991). Complications of indwelling venous access lines in the pediatric hematology patients: A prospective comparison of external venous catheters and subcutaneous ports. *Am J Pediatr Hematol Oncol*, 13(2):130-136.

Jacobs, W.R., & Zaroukian, M.H. (1991). Coughing and central venous catheter dislodgement. *JPEN*, 15(4).

Jarrd, M.M., Olsen, C.M., & Freeman, J.B. (1980). Daily dressing change effects on skin flora beneath subclavian catheter dressings during total parenteral nutrition. *JPEN*, 4(4):391-392.

Johnson, B.H. & Rypins,E.B.(1990). Single-lumen vs double-lumen catheters for total parenteral nutrition. *Arch Surg*, 125:990-992.

Kamal, G.D. et al. (1991). Reduced intravascular catheter infection by antibiotic bonding. A prospective, randomized, controlled trial. *JAMA*, May 8; 265(18): 2364-2368.

Kandt, K.A..(1991). An implantable venous access device for children. *Am J Mater Child Nurs*, 16(2):88-91.

Laffer, U. et al. (1991). Surgical experiences with 191 implanted venous Port-a-Cath systems. *Recent Results Cancer Res*, 121:189-197.

Landers, S. et al.(1991). Factors associated with umbilical catheter-related sepsis in neonates. *AJDC*, 145:675-680.

Lawson, M. (1991). Partial occlusion of indwelling central venous catheters, *JIN*, 14(3):157-159.

Lawson, M. (1982) The use of urokinase to restore the patency of occluded central venous catheters, American Journal of Intravenous Therapy and Clincial Nutrition, 29-32.

Lindblad, B. (1982) Thromboembolic complications and central venous catheters, *Lancet,* 2:936-937.

Lum, P. and Soski, M. (1989) Management of malpositioned central venous catheters, *JIN, 121*(6):356-365.

Maki, D.G.(1989). Risk factors for nosocomial infection in intensive care. *Arch Inter Med, 149*:30-35.

Maki, D.G. & Ringer, M. (1991). Risk factors for infusion-related phlebitis with small peripheral venous catheters. *Ann Intern Med, 114*: 845-854.

McKee, J.M., et al (1989). Complications of intravenous therapy: a randomized study–teflon vs vialon. *JIN, 12*(5):288-295.

Messing, B., Peitra-Cohen, S., Debure, A., et al. (1988). Antibiotic-lock technique: A new approach to optimal therapy for catheter-related sepsis in home-parenteral nutrition. *JPEN, 12*:185-189.

Miller, S.J., Dickerson, R.N., Mullen, J.L., Graziani, A.A., & Muscari, E.A. (1990). Antibiotic therapy of catheter infections in patients receiving home parenteral nutrition. *JPEN, 14*:143-147.

Mirro, J. et al.(1990). A comparison of placement techniques and complications of internalized catheters and implantable port use in children with cancer. *J Ped Surg, 25*(1):120-124.

Monturo, C.A., Dickerson, R.N., & Mullen, J.L.(1990). Efficacy of thrombolytic therapy for occlusion of long-term catheters, *JPEN, 14*:312-314.

Moosa, H.H.et al.(1991).Complications of indwelling central venous catheters in bone marrow transplant recipients. *Surg Gynecol Obstet, 172*(4):275-279.

Norwood,S. et al.(1991). Catheter-related infections and associated septicemia. *Chest, 99*:968-975.

Pennington, C.R. (1990). Management of catheter occlusion. *JPEN, 14*:551.

Pessa, M.E. & Howard, R.J. (1985). Complications of Hickman-Broviac catheters. *Surg Gynec & Obst, 161*:257-260.

Petrosino, B., Becker,H., & Christian, B. (1988). Infection rates in central venous catheter dressings. *ONF, 15*(6):709-717.

Putterman, C.(1990).Central venous catheter related sepsis: a clinical review. *Resuscitation 20*:1-16.

Rasor, J.S.(1991). Review of catheter-related infection rates: Comparison of conventional catheter materials with Aquavene®. *JAVAN. 1*(3):8.

Schmid, L. et al (1990). An open prospective trial to compare the hematological and biochemical routine laboratory result from a peripheral arm vein and from a fully implanted venous drug delivery device (letter). *Ann Oncol. 1*(1):82.

Schmidt-Sommerfield,E. et al (1990). Catheter-related complications in 35 children and adolescents with gastrointestinal disease on home parenteral nutrition. *JPEN. 14*(2):148-151.

Schropp, K.P., Ginn-Pease, M.E., & King, D.R. (1988). Catheter-related sepsis: A review of the experience with Broviac and Hickman catheters. *Nutrition, 4*:195-200.

Schulman, R.J., Reed, T., Pitre, D. et al (1988). Use of hydrochloric acid to clear obstructed central venous catheters. *JPEN, 12*(2):90-92.

Schulmeister, L.(1989). Needle dislodgements from implanted venous access devices; inpatient and outpatient experiences, *JIN, 12*(2):90-92.

Scott, W.L. (1988). Complication associated with central venous catheters. *Chest, 94*:1221-1224.

Segura, M. et al (1990). Assessment of a new hub design and semiquantitative catheter culture method using an in vivo experimental model of catheter sepsis. *J Clin Microbiol, 28*(11):1551-1554.

Smith,S. et al. (1991). Maintenance of patency of indwelling central venous catheters: Is heparin necessary? *Am J. Pediatr Hematol Oncol, 13* (2):141-143.

Stennet, D.J., Gerwick,W.H.,Egging,P.K., et al (1988). Precipitate analysis from an indwelling total parenteral nutrition catheter. *JPEN, 12*(1):88-92.

Syndman, D.R. et al. (1990). Nosocomial sepsis associated with interleukin-2. *Annals of Int Med, 112*:102-107.

Testerman, E.J. (1991).Restoring patency of central venous catheters obstructed by mineral precipitation using hydrochloric acid. *JVAN, 1*(1):22.

Testerman, J. (1991) Restoring patency of central venous catheters obstructed by mineral precipitation using hydrochloric acid, *JVAN* 1 (2):22.

Ullman, R.F.(1990). Colonization and bacteremia related to duration of triple-lumen intravascular catheter placement. *J Infect Control, 18*:201-207.

VanHoff, J.,Berg, A.T. & Seashore, J.H. (1990). The effect of right atrial catheters on infectious complications of chemotherapy in children. *J Clin Onc, 8*(7):1255-1261.

Viall, C. (1990). Daily access of implanted ports: implications for patient education. *JIM, 13*(5):294-296.

Wickham, R.S. (1990). Advances in venous devices and nursing management strategies. *Nurs Clin of North Am, 25*(2):345-363.

Wiernikowski, J.T. et al(1991). Bacterial colonization of tunneled right atrial catheters in pediatric oncology: A comparison of sterile saline and bacteriostatic saline flush solutions. *Am J Pediatr Hematol Oncol,* *13*(2):137-140.

Yagupsky, P. & Nolte, F. (1990). Quantitative aspects of septicemia. *J Clin Microbiol, 3*(3):269-279.

CHEMOTHERAPEUTIC AGENTS MOST FREQUENTLY GIVEN IN THE HOME

Vivian West, RN, BSN, MBA
National Director of Nursing, NMC Homecare, Waltham, MA

CHEMOTHERAPEUTIC AGENTS MOST FREQUENTLY GIVEN IN THE HOME

Vivian West, RN, BSN, MBA
National Director of Nursing NMC Homecare
Waltham, Massachusetts

The administration of chemotherapy outside the hospital setting is becoming more the norm than the exception. It is therefore important that nursing care plans recognize the different side effects that can be caused by the different chemotherapeutic agents. The following drug information is generic but the care plans specifically relate to the side effects pertinent to these drugs. The care plans utilize a portion of NMC Homecare's standardized care plans.

All information is adapted from *Cancer Chemotherapy: A Nursing Process Approach* by Barton Burke, Wilkes, Berg, Bean, and Ingwersen published by Jones & Bartlett Publishers, Inc. Boston, Massachusetts (1991) and *Chemotherapy Care Plans: Designs for Nursing Care* by Barton Burke, Wilkes, and Ingwersen published by Jones & Bartlett Publishers, Inc. Boston, Massachusetts (1992).

Included are care plans for the seven chemotherapeutic agents most commonly administered by NMC Homecare nurses.

DRUG

Cyclophosphamide (Cytoxan, Endoxan, Endoxana, Neosar)

Class: Alkylating agent

MECHANISM OF ACTION

Causes cross-linkage in DNA strands thus preventing DNA synthesis and cell division. Cell cycle phase nonspecific.

METABOLISM

Inactive until converted by microsomes in liver and serum enzymes (phosphamidases). Both cyclophosphamide and its metabolites are excreted by the kidneys.

Plasma half-life: 6-12 hours, with 25% drug excreted by 8 hours. Prolonged plasma half-life in patients with renal failure results in increased myelosuppression.

DOSAGE/RANGE

400mg/m² IV x 5 days

100 mg/m² PO x 14 days

500-1500 mg/m² IV q 3-4 weeks

DRUG PREPARATION

Dilute vials with sterile water. Shake well. Allow solution to clear if lyophilised preparation is not used.

Do not use solution unless crystals are fully dissolved. Available in 25 and 50 mg tablets.

DRUG ADMINISTRATION

PO use – administer in morning or early afternoon to allow adequate excretion time. Should be taken with meals.

IV use – for doses greater than 500 mg, pre- and posthydration to total 500-3000 ml is needed to ensure adequate urine output and avoid hemorrhagic cystitis. Administer drug over at least 20 min for doses greater than 500 mg.

Solution is stable for 24 hours at room temperature, 6 days if refrigerated.

Rapid infusion may result in dizziness, nasal stuffiness, rhinorrhea, sinus congestion during or soon after infusion.

SPECIAL CONSIDERATIONS

Metabolic and leukopenic toxicity is increased by simultaneous administration of barbiturates, corticosteroids, phenytoin, and sulfonamides.

Activity and toxicity of both cyclophosphamide and the specific drug may be altered by allopurinol, chloroquine, phenothiazides, potassium iodide, chloramphenicol, imipramine, vitamin A, warfarin, succinylcholine, digoxin, thiazide diuretics. Test urine for occult blood.

High-dose cyclophosphamide therapy may require catheterization and constant bladder irrigation.

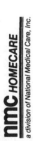

PATENT CARE PLAN

nmc *HOMECARE*
a division of National Medical Care, Inc.

Diagnosis:

Therapy: Chemotherapy (Cyclophosphamide)

Nursing Diagnosis	Goals	Interventions
1. Altered nutrition: less than body requirements related to		
A. Nausea and vomiting • *Nausea and vomiting begin 2-4 hrs after dose, peak in 12 hrs, and may last 24 hrs*	1. Pt will be without nausea and vomiting 2. Nausea and vomiting, if they occur, will be minimal	1. Premedicate with antiemetics and continue prophylactically x 24 hrs to prevent nausea and vomiting, at least for first treatment
B. Anorexia • *Commonly occurs*	3. Pt will maintain baseline weight +/- 5%	2. Encourage small, frequent feedings of favorite foods, especially high-calorie, high-protein foods (bland if pt has N/V) 3. Encourage use of spices as tolerated with anorexia 4. Weekly weights 5. Nutritional consultation as needed
C. Stomatitis • *Mild*	4. Oral mucous membranes will remain intact without infection	6. Teach pt oral assessment and oral hygiene regimen; and encourage pt to report early stomatitis
D. Diarrhea • *Infrequent and mild*	5. Pt will have minimal diarrhea	7. Encourage pt to report onset of diarrhea, and administer, or teach pt to self administer, antidiarrheal medications

E. Hepatotoxicity • *Rare*	6. Early hepatoxicity will be identified	8. Monitor LFTs, i.e., alkaline phosphatase and bilirubin, periodically during treatment for any elevations • *Dose modifications may be necessary if elevation occurs*
2. Infection and bleeding related to bone marrow depression • *Leukopenia nadir 7-14 days with recovery in 1-2 weeks* • *Less frequent thrombocytopenia* • *Mild anemia* • *Potent immunosuppressant*	1. Pt will be without infection or bleeding 2. S/s of infection or bleeding, if they occur, will be identified early	1. Monitor CBC, platelet count prior to drug administration and monitor for s/s of infection and bleeding 2. Instruct pt in self-assessment of s/s of infection and bleeding • *Dose reduction often necessary (35-50%) if compromised bone marrow function*
3. Potential for injury related to A. Acute water intoxication(SIADH) • *May occur with high-dose administration (>50 mg/kg)* B. Second malignancy (bladder CA, acute leukemia) • *Prolonged therapy may cause bladder cancer (related to local toxicity of drug metabolites) and acute leukemia (related to prolonged bone marrow toxicity)*	1. SIADH will be identified early 2. Malignancy, if it occurs, will be identified early	1. If high-dose cytoxan administered, monitor serum sodium, osmolality, and urine electrolytes and osmolality 2. QD weights 3. Strictly monitor I/O and total body balance 4. Water restrictions as ordered 5. Pts receiving prolonged therapy should be screened *(continued)*

(continued)

Diagnosis:

Therapy: Chemotherapy (Cyclophosphamide)

Nursing Diagnosis	Goals	Interventions
4. Altered urinary elimination, related to hemorrhagic cystitis • *Metabolites of cyclophosphamide, if allowed to accumulate in bladder, irritate bladder wall capillaries causing hemorrhagic cystitis* • *Sterile chemical cystitis occurs in 5%–10% of pts* • *Evidenced by hematuria, gross or microscopic(>20rbc)* • *Is preventable* • *Another potential side effect is bladder fibrosis*	1. Pt will be without hemorrhagic cystitis	1. Monitor BUN and creatinine prior to drug dose • *Drug is excreted by kidneys* 2. Provide or instruct pt in hydration of at least 3 L of fluid/day 3. Encourage voiding to empty bladder at least q 2-3 hours, and at bedtime 4. Assess pt for signs of and instruct pt to report signs of hematuria, urinary frequency, dysuria 5. Instruct pt to take cyclophosphamide early in day to prevent accumulation of drug in the bladder
5. Alteration in cardiac output, related to high-dose cyclophosphamide • *Cardiomyopathy may occur with high doses; also, potentiates cardiotoxicity of doxorubicin (Adriamycin)*	1. Early s/s of cardiomyopathy will be identified	1. Assess for s/s of cardiomyopathy 2. Discuss need for gated blood pool scan with MD 3. Assess quality and regularity of heartbeat 4. Instruct pt to report dyspnea, shortness of breath

Nursing Diagnosis	Expected Outcomes	Nursing Interventions
6. Potential for impaired gas exchange, related to pulmonary toxicity • *Rare, but may occur with prolonged, high-dose therapy or continuous low-dose therapy* • *Appears as interstitial pneumonitis: onset is insidious* • *May respond to steroids*	1. Early s/s of pulmonary toxicity will be identified	1. If pt is receiving high-dose or continuous low-dose cyclophosphamide A. Assess for s/s of pulmonary dysfunction B. Discuss pulmonary function studies to be performed periodically with MD C. Assess lung sounds prior to drug administration D. Instruct pt to report cough or dyspnea
7. Altered body image related to A. Alopecia • *Occurs in 30-50% of pts, especially with IV dosing* • *Some degree of hair loss expected in all patients* • *Begins after 3+ weeks and may grow back while on therapy* • *May be slight to diffuse thinning* B. Changes in nails, skin • *Hyperpigmentation of nails and skin, transverse ridging of nails ("banding") may occur*	1. Pt will verbalize feelings re: hair loss, and identify strategies to cope with change in body image 2. Pt will verbalize feelings re: changes in nail or skin color or texture, and identify strategies to cope with change in body image	1. Assess pt for s/s of hair loss 2. Discuss with pt impact of hair loss, and strategies to minimize distress; i.e., wig, scarf, cap • *Begin discussion before therapy has been initiated* 3. Assess pt for changes in skin, nails 4. Discuss with pt impact of changes, and strategies to minimize distress; i.e., wearing nail polish (women), long sleeved tops
8. Potential for sexual dysfunction • *Drug is mutagenic and teratogenic* • *Testicular atrophy sometimes occurs with reversible oligo and azoospermia* • *Amenorrhea often occurs in females* • *Drug is excreted in breast milk*	1. Pt and significant other will understand need for contraception 2. Pt and significant other will identify strategies to cope with sexual dysfunction	1. As appropriate, explore with pt and significant other issues of reproductive and sexuality patterns, and the impact chemotherapy will have on these activities 2. Discuss strategies to preserve sexual and reproductive health (i.e., sperm banking, contraception)

DRUG

5-Fluorouracil (Fluorouracil, Adrudil, 5-FU, Efudex (topical))

Class: Pyrimidine Antimetabolite

MECHANISM

Acts as a "false" pyrimidine, inhibiting the formation of an enzyme (thymidine synthetase) necessary for the synthesis of DNA. Also incorporated into RNA, causing abnormal synthesis. Methotrexate given prior to 5-Fluorouracil results in synergism and enhanced efficacy.

METABOLISM

Metabolized by the liver, most is excreted as respiratory CO_2; remainder is excreted by the kidneys.

Plasma half-life is 20 minutes.

DOSAGE/RANGE

12-15mg/kg IV once per week or 12 mg/kg IV every day x 5 days every 4 weeks or 500 mg/m² every week or every week x 5.

Hepatic infusion: 22 mg/kg in 100 ml. D_5W infused into hepatic artery over 8 hours for 5-21 consecutive days.

Head and neck: 1000 mg/m² x 4-5 days as continuous infusion.

DRUG PREPARATION

No dilution required. Can be added to NS or D_5W.

Store at room temperature; protect from light. Solution should be clear; if crystals do not disappear after holding vial under hot water, discard vial.

DRUG ADMINSTRATION

Given IV push or bolus (slow drip), or as continuous infusion.

Topical: as cream.

SPECIAL CONSIDERATIONS

Cutaneous side effects occur, e.g., skin sensitivity to sun, splitting of fingernails, dry, flaky skin, and hyperpigmentation on face, palms of hands.

Patients who have had adrenalectomy may need higher doses of prednisone while receiving 5-FU or dose of 5-FU may be reduced in postadrenalectomy patients.

Reduce dose in patients with compromised hepatic, renal, or bone marrow function and malnutrition.

Inspect solution for precipitate prior to continous infusion.

When given with cimetidine there are increased pharmacologic effects of fluorouracil.

When given with thiazide diuretics there is increased risk of myelosuppression.

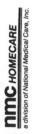

nmc HOMECARE
a division of National Medical Care, Inc.

Diagnosis:

Therapy: Chemotherapy (5-Flurouracil)

Nursing Diagnosis	Goals	Interventions

1. Altered nutrition: less than body requirements related to
 	
A. Nausea and vomiting
• *Occurs occasionally, may last 2-3 days, usually preventable with antiemetics*
 	
B. Stomatitis
• *Onset 5-8 days*
• *May herald severe bone marrow depression*
• *Is an indication to interrupt therapy*
 	
C. Diarrhea
• *Indication to interrupt treatment*
• *May occur with esophagopharyngitis - sore throat with dysphagia*
	1. Pt will be without nausea or vomiting
	2. Nausea and vomiting, if they occur, will be minimal
	
	3. Oral mucous membranes will remain intact and free of infection
	
	4. Pt will have minimal diarrhea
	5. Early s/s of esophagopharyngitis will be identified and treated
		1. Premedicate with antiemetics and continue prophylactically x 24 hrs to prevent nausea and vomiting, at least with the first treatment
		2. Encourage small, frequent feedings of cool, bland foods and liquids
		3. Assess for s/s of fluid and electrolyte imbalance
		4. Assess mouth prior to each dose and report stomatitis to MD
		   • *Stomatitis is sometimes preceded by a beefy, painful tongue or small, shallow ulcers on the inner lip*
		5. Teach pt oral assessment and mouth care
		6. Encourage pt to report onset of diarrhea, and
		   A. Administer or teach pt to self-administer antidiarrheal medication
		   B. Guaiac all stools
		   C. Encourage adequate hydration
		   D. Assess pt for sore throat, dysphagia, and treat with topical anesthetics

Nursing Diagnosis / Rationale	Expected Outcomes	Nursing Interventions
2. Infection and bleeding, related to bone marrow depression • *Common* • *Neutropenia, thrombocytopenia are most significant* • *Nadir 7-14 days after first dose*	1. Pt will be without infection or bleeding 2. S/s of infection or bleeding, if they occur, will be identified early	1. Monitor CBC, platelet count prior to drug administration 2. Instruct pt in self-assessment of s/s of infection and bleeding
3. Alteration in skin integrity, related to A. Alopecia • *More common with 5-day courses of treatment. Uncommon with 1-day courses* • *Diffuse thinning, loss of eyelashes and eyebrows* B. Changes in nails and skin • *Nail loss and brittle cracking of nails may occur* • *Photosensitivity/photophobia may occur* • *Maculopapular rash sometimes occurs on the extremities and trunk (rarely serious)* • *Chemical phlebitis may occur during continuous infusions related to high pH of drug*	1. Pt will verbalize feelings re: hair loss, and identify strategies to cope with change in body image 2. Pt will verbalize feelings re: changes in nails and skin and will identify strategies to cope with changes in body image	1. Assess pt for s/s of hair loss 2. Discuss with pt impact of alterations, and strategies to minimize distress (e.g., wearing nail polish for women or long sleeve tops) 3. Instruct pt in importance of staying out of sun or wearing sunscreen if sun exposure is unavoidable 4. Assess skin for rash or other changes. Report changes to MD. Pt may need antihistamines or steroids
4. Alteration in sensory perception • *Occasional cerebellar ataxia (reversible when drug is discontinued)* • *Somnolence* • *Ocular changes: conjunctivitis, increased lacrimation, photophobia, oculomotor dysfunction, blurred vision* • *Occasional euphoria*	1. Early neurological changes will be identified 2. Pt will identify strategies for coping with neurological changes	1. Assess cerebellar function prior to each treatment 2. Teach pt safety precautions 3. Assess pt for ocular changes. Report changes

DRUG

Vinblastine (Velban)

Class: Plant alkaloid extracted from the periwinkle plant (Vinca rosea)

MECHANISM

Drug binds to microtubular proteins thus arresting mitosis during metaphase; may inhibit RNA, DNA, and protein synthesis. Active in S and M Phases (cell cycle phase specific).

METABOLISM

About 10% of drug is excreted in feces. Vinblastine is partially metabolized by the liver. Minimal amount of the drug is excreted in urine and bile. Dose modification may be necessary in the presence of hepatic failure.

DOSAGE/RANGE

0.1 mg/kg; 6mg/m² IV weekly: continuous infusion 1.4-1.8 mg/day x 5 days.

DRUG PREPARATION

Available in 10-mg vials. Store in refrigerator until use.

DRUG ADMINISTRATION

Intravenous. This drug is a vesicant. Give through the sidearm of a running IV so as to avoid extravasation which can lead to ulceration, pain, and necrosis. Be sure to check nursing procedure for administration of a vesicant.

SPECIAL CONSIDERATIONS

Drug is a *vesicant.* Give through a running IV to avoid *extravasation.*

Dose modification may be necessary in the presence of hepatic failure.

Decreased pharmacologic effects of phenytoin when given with this drug.

Increases cellular uptake of methotrexate by certain malignant cells when administered sequentially, but less so than vincristine.

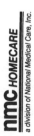

nmc HOMECARE
a division of National Medical Care, Inc.

Diagnosis:

Therapy: Chemotherapy (vinblastine)

Nursing Diagnosis	Goals	Interventions
1. Potential for infection and bleeding related to bone marrow depression (BMD) • *May cause severe BMD* • *Nadir 4–10 days* • *Neutrophils greatly affected* • *In pts with prior XRT or chemotherapy, thrombocytopenia may be severe*	1. Pt will be without infection or bleeding 2. S/s of infection or bleeding, if they occur, will be identified early	1. Monitor CBC, platelet count prior to drug administration 2. Instruct pt in self-assessment of s/s of infection or bleeding 3. Administer red cell, platelet transfusions as ordered
2. Potential for sensory/perceptual alterations • *Occur less frequently than with vincristine* • *Occur in pts receiving prolonged or high-dose therapy* • *Symptoms: paresthesias, peripheral neuropathy, depression, headache, malaise, jaw pain, urinary retention, tachycardia, orthostatic hypotension, seizures* • *Rare ocular changes: diplopia, ptosis, photophobia, oculomotor dysfunction, optic neuropathy*	1. Sensory/perceptual changes will be identified early 2. Dysfunction will be minimized 3. Discomfort will be minimized	1. Assess sensory/perceptual changes prior to each drug dose • *This is especially important if dose is high (> 10 mg) or pt is receiving prolonged therapy* 2. Notify MD of alterations 3. Discuss impact changes have had with pt, and strategies to minimize dysfunction and decrease distress

3. Altered bowel elimination due to constipation • *Constipation results from neurotoxicity (central) and is less common than with vincristine* • *Risk factors: high dose (>20 mg/m²)* • *May lead to adynamic ileus, abdominal pain*	1. Constipation will be prevented 2. Early s/s of ileus will be identified	1. Assess bowel elimination pattern with each drug dose (especially if dose > 20 mg) 2. Teach pt to promote bowel elimination by increasing fluids, (3 L/day), high fiber, bulky foods, exercise, stool softeners • *Suggest laxative if unable to move bowels at least once a day* 3. Instruct pt to report abdominal pain
4. Altered nutrition: less than body requirements related to A. Nausea and vomiting • *Rarely occur*	1. Pt will be without nausea and vomiting 2. Nausea and vomiting, if they occur, will be minimal	1. Premedicate with antiemetics and continue prophylactically x 24 hrs to prevent nausea and vomiting, at least for the first treatment 2. Encourage small, frequent feedings of cool, bland foods and liquids 3. Assess for symptoms of fluid and electro-lyte imbalance: monitor daily weights
B. Stomatitis • *Occurs occasionally, but may be severe*	3. Oral mucous membranes will remain intact and without infection	4. Teach pt oral assessment and oral hygiene regimens, and encourage pt to report early stomatitis
C. Diarrhea • *Occasional, infrequent, and mild*	4. Pt will have minimal diarrhea	5. Encourage pt to report onset of diarrhea, administer or teach pt to self-administer antidiarrheal medication, and teach diet modification

(continued)

Diagnosis:

Therapy: Chemotherapy (vinblastine)

(continued)

Nursing Diagnosis	Goals	Interventions

5. Potential for altered body image related to
 	
A. Alopecia
  • *Reversible and mild*
  • *Occurs in 45%–50% of pts receiving drug*
 	
B. Extravasation
  • *Drug is a potent vesicant and can cause irritation and necrosis if infiltrated*
	1. Pt will verbalize feelings regarding hair loss
	2. Pt will identify strategies to cope with changes in body image
	
	3. Extravasation will be avoided
	4. Skin will heal completely if extravasation occurs
		1. Explore with pt response to actual hair loss and plan strategies to minimize distress, i.e., wig, scarf, cap
		
		2. Administer vesicant through newly cannulated freely flowing IV, constantly monitoring IV site and pt response
		  • *Nurse should be THOROUGHLY familiar with institutional policy and procedure for administration of a vesicant agent*
		  • *Careful technique is used during venipuncture*
		  • *If a vesicant drug is administered as a continuous infusion, drug must be given through a patent central line*
		  • *If extravasation is suspected:*
		    a. Stop drug administration
		    b. Aspirate any residual drug and blood from IV tubing, IV catheter/needle, and IV site if possible
		    c. If drug infiltration is suspected, manufacturer suggests the following after withdrawing any remaining drug from IV: local instillation of hyaluronidase, apply moderate heat
		    d. Assess site regularly for pain, progression of erythema, induration, and for evidence of necrosis

		• When in doubt about whether drug is infiltrating, TREAT AS AN INFILTRATION • Teach pt to assess site and notify MD if condition worsens • Arrange next clinic visit for assessment of site depending on drug, amount infiltrated, extent of potential injury, and pt variables • Document in pt's record as per institutional policy and procedure
C. Rash • *Uncommon*	5. Pt will identify strategies to cope with rash	3. Assess impact of rash on pt: body image, comfort, and treat symptomatically
6. Potential for sexual dysfunction • *Drug is possibly teratogenic* • *Likely to cause azoospermia in men*	1. Pt and significant other will identify strategies to cope with sexual dysfunction	1. As appropriate, explore with pt and significant other issues of reproductive and sexuality patterns and anticipated impact chemotherapy may have 2. Discuss strategies to preserve sexual health (e.g., sperm banking)

DRUG

Vincristine (Oncovin)

Class: Plant alkaloid extracted from the periwinkle plant (Vinca rosea)

MECHANISM

Drug binds to microtubular proteins thus arresting mitosis during metaphase. Cell cycle phase specific in M and S phases.

METABOLISM

The primary route for excretion is via the liver with about 70% of the drug being excreted in feces and bile.

These metabolites are a result of hepatic metabolism and biliary excretion. A small amount is excreted in the urine. Dose modification may be necessary in the presence of hepatic failure.

DOSAGE/RANGE

0.4-1.4 mg/m^2 weekly (initially limited to 2 mg per dose).

DRUG PREPARATION

Supplied in 1-mg, 2-mg and 5-mg vials. Refrigerate vials until use.

DRUG ADMINISTRATION

Intravenous. This drug is a vesicant. Give through running IV to avoid extravasation which can lead to ulceration, pain, and necrosis. Be sure to check nursing procedure for administration of a vesicant.

SPECIAL CONSIDERATIONS

Drug is a *vesicant*. Give through a running IV to avoid *extravasation*.

Dose modification may be necessary in the presence of hepatic failure.

Decreased bioavailability of digoxin when given with this drug.

Increased cellular uptake of methotrexate by some malignant cells when given sequentially.

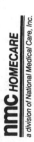

Diagnosis:

Therapy: Chemotherapy (vincristine)

Nursing Diagnosis	Goals	Interventions

1. Potential for sensory/perceptual alteration related to
 	
A. Peripheral neuropathies
  • *Peripheral neuropathies occur as a result of toxicity to nerve fibers*
  • *Absent deep tendon reflexes*
  • *Numbness, weakness, myalgias, cramping*
  • *Late severe motor difficulties*
  • *Reversal or discontinuance of therapy necessary*
  • *Increased risk in elderly*
 	
B. Cranial nerve damage and other nerve involvement
  • *Cranial nerve dysfunction may occur (rare)*
  • *Jaw pain (trigeminal neuralgia)*
  • *Diplopia*
  • *Vocal cord paresis*
  • *Mental depression*
  • *Metallic taste*
	1. Sensory and perceptual changes will be identified early
	2. Dysfunction will be minimized
	3. Discomfort will be minimized
	
	4. Symptoms of nerve dysfunction will be identified early
		1. Assess sensory and perceptual changes prior to each drug dose (presence of numbness or tingling of fingertips or toes)
		2. Assess for loss of tendon reflexes (foot drop, slapping gait)
		3. Assess for motor difficulties (clumsiness of hands, difficulty climbing stairs, difficulty buttoning shirt, walking on heels)
		4. Notify MD of alterations
		  • *Discuss holding drug if loss of deep tendon reflexes occur*
		5. Discuss with pt impact alterations have had, and strategies to minimize dysfunction and decrease distress
		6. Discuss with pt type of alteration: memory, sensory/perceptual changes, temporary and reversible when drug stopped
		7. Assess pt for s/s of nerve dysfunction before each dose and notify MD of any changes

C. Constipation
- *Autonomic neuropathy may lead to constipation and paralytic ileus*
- *A concurrent use of vincristine, narcotic analgesics, or cholinergic medication may increase risk of constipation*

5. Constipation will be prevented
6. Early s/s of paralytic ileus will be identified

8. Assess bowel elimination pattern prior to each chemotherapy administration
9. Teach pt to include bulky and high fiber foods in diet, increase fluids to 3 L/day, and exercise moderately to promote elimination
10. Suggest stool softeners
11. Teach pt to use laxative if unable to move bowels at least once every 2 days
12. Instruct pt to report abdominal pain

2. Potential for impaired skin integrity related to
A. Alopecia
- *Complete hair loss occurs in 12%–45% of pts*
- *Both men and women are at risk for body image disturbance*
- *Hair will grow back*

1. Pt will verbalize feelings about hair loss and identify strategies to cope with changes in body image

1. Discuss with pt anticipated impact of hair loss; suggest wig or toupee as appropriate prior to actual hair loss
2. Explore with pt response to hair loss, if it occurs, and strategies to minimize distress, i.e., wig, scarf, cap

B. Dermatitis
- *Uncommon*

2. Pt will identify coping strategies

3. Discuss strategies to minimize distress if dermatitis develops

C. Extravasation
- *Drug is potent vesicant causing irritation and necrosis if infiltrated*

3. Extravasation will be avoided
4. Skin will heal completely if drug is extravasated

4. Administer vesicant through newly cannulated freely flowing IV, constantly monitoring IV site and pt response
- *If a vesicant drug is administered as a continuous infusion, drug must be given through a patent central line*
- *If extravasation is suspected:*
  a. Stop drug administered
  b. Aspirate any residual drug and blood from IV tubing, IV catheter/needle, and IV site if possible
  c. If drug infiltration is suspected, manufacturer suggests the following after withdrawing any remaining drug from IV: local instillation of hyaluronidase, apply moderate heat
  d. Assess site regularly for pain, progression of erythema, induration, and for evidence of necrosis

(continued)

Diagnosis: **Therapy:** Chemotherapy (vincristine) *(continued)*

Nursing Diagnosis	Goals	Interventions
		• *When in doubt about whether drug is infiltrating, TREAT AS AN INFILTRATION* • *Teach pt to assess site and notify MD if condition worsens* • *Arrange next clinic visit for assessment of site depending on drug, amount infiltrated, extent of potential injury, and pt variables* • *Document in pt's record as per institutional policy and procedure*
3. Potential for infection and bleeding related to bone marrow depression • *Rare myelosuppression, mild when it occurs* • *May have depression of platelets over time requiring transfusion* • *Nadir 10-14 days after treatment begins*	1. Pt will be without bleeding or infection 2. S/s of bleeding or infection, if they occur, will be detected early	1. Monitor WBC, Hct, platelets prior to drug administration
4. Potential for sexual dysfunction • *Impotence may occur related to neurotoxicity*	1. Pt and significant other will identify strategies to cope with sexual dysfunction	1. As appropriate, explore with pt and significant other issues of reproductive and sexuality patterns and impact chemotherapy may have 2. Discuss strategies to preserve sexual health, i.e., alternative expressions of sexuality 3. Reassure pt that impotence, if it occurs, is usually temporary, and reversible after drug discontinuance

DRUG

Doxorubicin hydrochloride (Adriamycin, Rubex)

Class: Anthracycline antibiotic isolated from streptomycin products, in particular from the rhodomycin products.

MECHANISM OF ACTION

Antitumor antibiotic- no clearly defined mechanism. Binds directly to DNA base pairs (intercalates) and inhibit DNA and DNA- dependent RNA synthesis, as well as protein synthesis. Cell cycle specific for S-phase.

METABOLISM

Excretion of drug predominates in the liver; renal clearance is minor. Alteration in liver function requires modification of doses, whereas with renal failure there is no need to alter doses. Drug excreted through urine and may discolor urine from 1-48 hours after administration.

DOSAGE/RANGE

30-75 mg/m^2 IV every 3-4 weeks.

20-45 mg/m^2 IV for 3 consecutive days.

For bladder instillation: 3-60mg/m^2.

For intraperitoneal instillation: 40 mg in 2 L dialysate (no heparin).

Continuous infusion: varies with individual protocol.

DRUG PREPARATION

Drug will form a precipitate if mixed with heparin or 5-fluorouracil. Dilute with Sodium Chloride (preservative free) to produce 2 mg/mL concentration.

DRUG ADMINISTRATION

IV. This drug is a potent vesicant. Give through a running IV to avoid extravasation which can lead to ulceration, pain, and necrosis. Be sure to check nursing procedure for administration of a vesicant.

SPECIAL CONSIDERATIONS

Drug is a potent *vesicant*. Give through a running IV to avoid *extravasation* and tissue necrosis.

Give through central line if drug is to be given by continuous infusion.

Nausea and vomiting is dose related. Occurs in 50% of patients. Begins 1-3 hours after administration.

Causes discoloration of urine (from pink to red for up to 48 hours).

Skin changes: may cause "recall phenomenon" - recalls reaction to previously irradiated tissue.

Potent myelosuppressive agent causes gastrointestinal toxicites: mucositis, esophagitis, and diarrhea.

Cardiac Toxicity- dose limit at 550 mg/m^2. Patients may exhibit irreversible congestive heart failure. May see acute toxicity in hours or days after administration. This is unrelated to cumulative dose and may manifest symptoms of pump or conduction dysfunction. Rarely, transient EKG abnormalities, CHF, pericardial effusions (whole syndrome referred to as myocarditis-pericarditis syndrome) may occur, which may lead to demise of patient.

Vein discoloration.

Increased pigmentation in black patients.

When given with barbiturates there is increased plasma clearance of doxorubicin.

When given with cyclophosphamide there is risk of hemorrhage and cardiotoxicity.

When given with mitomycin there is increased risk of cardiotoxicity.

There is decreased oral bioavailability of digoxin when given together.

When given with mercaptopurine there is increased risk of hepatotoxicity.

nmc *HOMECARE*
a division of National Medical Care, Inc.

Diagnosis:

Therapy: Chemotherapy (doxorubicin)

Nursing Diagnosis	Goals	Interventions

1. Potential for infection and bleeding related to bone marrow depression
• *Nadir 10-14 days with recovery 15-21 days*
• *Myelosuppression may be severe: overall incidence 60-80%, less common with weekly dosing*
	1. Pt will be without s/s of infection or bleeding
	2. S/s of infection or bleeding, if they occur, will be detected early.
		1. Instruct pt in self-assessment of s/s of infection and bleeding
		  • *Dose reduction may be necessary, discuss with MD*
		  • *Transfuse with red cells and platelets per MD order*
		2. Monitor CBC, platelet count prior to drug administration

2. Potential for alteration in nutrition, due to
 	
A. Nausea and vomiting
  • *Moderate to severe; 50% incidence as single agent with increased incidence in combination with Cytoxan*
  • *Onset 1-3 hours after drug administration, lasting up to 24 hours*
 	
B. Anorexia
  • *Occurs frequently*
 	
C. Stomatitis
  • *10% incidence of esophagitis*
	1. Pt will be without nausea and vomiting
	2. Nausea and vomiting, if they occur, will be minimal
	
	3. Pt will maintain baseline weight +/- 5%
	
	4. Oral mucous membrane will remain intact without infection
		1. Premedicate with antiemetics and continue prophylactically 24 hrs to prevent nausea and vomiting, at least first treatment
		2. Encourage small, frequent feedings of favorite foods, especially high-calorie, high-protein foods (cool, bland food & liquids if pt has N/V)
		3. Encourage use of spices as tolerated for anorexia
		4. Weekly weights
		5. Teach pt oral assessment and oral hygiene, and encourage pt to report early signs of stomatitis

(continued)

Diagnosis:

Therapy: Chemotherapy (doxorubicin)

(continued)

Nursing Diagnosis	Goals	Interventions

3. Potential for alteration in cardiac output
• *Acute: Pericarditis - myocarditis syndrome with nonspecific EKG changes (flat T-waves, ST, PVCs) during infusion or immediately after (non-life threatening)*
• *Cumulative dose cardiomyopathy: risk if dose >550mg/m² or >450 mg/m² receiving chest XRT or Cyotoxan*
	1. Early s/s of cardiomyopathy will be identified	1. Assess pt's baseline prior to beginning chemotherapy
		2. Assess quality and regularity of heartbeat
		3. Instruct pt to report dyspnea, shortness of breath
		  • *If pt is receiving cyclophosphamide in addition to doxorubicin assess for s/s of cardiomyopathy*
		  • *Cardiac evaluation on a regular basis*
		  • *Discuss gated blood pool scans with MD, baseline and periodically*

4. Potential for alteration in sexual function • *Drug is teratogenic and mutagenic*	1. Pt and significant other will understand need for contraception 2. Pt and significant other will identify strategies to cope with sexual dysfunction	1. As appropriate, explore with pt and significant other reproductive and sexuality patterns and impact chemotherapy will have 2. Discuss strategies to preserve sexuality and reproductive health (i.e. sperm banking, contraception)

5. Alteration in body image due to
  A. Alopecia
  • *Complete hair loss with 60-75 mg/m² dosing*
  • *Occurs 2-5 weeks after therapy begins*
  • *Regrowth usually begins a few months after drug is stopped*
	1. Pt will verbalize feelings re: hair loss and identify strategies to cope with change in body image	1. Assess pt for s/s of hair loss and discuss with pt impact of hair loss and strategies to minimize distress; i.e., wig, scarf, cap

B. Changes in nails and skin, radiation • *Nail beds and dermal creases (especially in black pts) become hyperpigmented* • *Reactivation of the erythema and skin damage of prior sites of skin irradiation* • *Erythematous streaking along vein during drug administration, often with urticaria and pruritis*	2. Pt will verbalize feelings re: changes in nail or skin color and texture, and identify strategies to cope with change in body image	2. Assess pt for changes in skin and nails and discuss with pt impact of changes and strategies to minimize distress; i.e., wearing nail polish (women) or long sleeve tops
6. Potential for alteration in skin integrity A. Extravasation • *Avoid extravasation as tissue necrosis may occur*	3. Extravasation, if it occurs, is detected early with early intervention, and skin and underlying tissue damage is minimized	3. Administer vesicant through newly cannulated freely flowing IV, constantly monitoring IV site and pt response • *If a vesicant drug is administered as a continuous infusion, drug must be given through a patent central line* • *If extravasation is suspected:* *a. Stop drug administration* *b. Aspirate any residual drug and blood from IV tubing, IV catheter/needle, and IV site if possible* *c. If drug infiltration is suspected, instill antidote into area of apparent infiltration, if antidote exists, as per MD orders and institutional policy and procedure. Apply cold or topical medication per MD order, and institutional policy and procedure* *d. Assess site regularly for pain, progression of erythema, induration, and for evidence of necrosis* • *When in doubt about whether drug is infiltrating, TREAT AS AN INFILTRATION* • *Teach pt to assess site and notify MD if condition worsens* • *Arrange next clinic visit for assessment of site depending on drug, amount infiltrated, extent of potential injury, and pt variables* • *Document in pt's record as per institutional policy and procedure*

DRUG

Cytarabine, Cytosine arabinoside (Ara-C, Cytosar-U, Arabinosyl Cytosine)

Class: Antimetabolite

MECHANISM OF ACTION

Antimetabolite (pyrimidine analogue) that is incorporated into DNA, slowing its synthesis and causing defects in the linkages of new DNA fragments. Also, cells exposed to cytarabine in the S phase reinitiate DNA synthesis when the drug is removed, resulting in erroneous duplications of the early portions of the DNA strands. Most effective when cells are undergoing rapid DNA synthesis.

METABOLISM

Inactivated by liver enzymes in biphasic manner: half-lives 10-15 minutes and 2-3 hours. Crosses the bloodbrain barrier with CSF concentration of 50% that of plasma. 70% of dose excreted in urine as Ara-U. 4%-10% excreted 12-24 hours after administration.

DOSAGE/RANGE

(varies depending upon disease)

Leukemia: 100 mg/m^2/day IV continuous infusion x 5-10 days

100 mg/m^2 every 12 hours x 1-3 weeks IV or SQ

Head and Neck: 1mg/kg every 12 hours x 5-7 days IV or SQ.

High Dose: 2-3 g/m^2 IV.

Differentiation: 10 mg/m^2 SQ every 12 hours x 15-21 days.

Intrathecal: 20-30 mg/m^2.

DRUG PREPARATION

100-mg vials: Add water with benzyl alcohol then dilute with NS or D$_5$W.

500-mg vials: Add water with benzyl alcohol then dilute with NS or D$_5$W.

For intrathecal use and high dose: Use preservative-free diluent.

Reconstituted drug is stable 48 hours at room temperature and 7 days refrigerated.

DRUG ADMINISTRATION (CYTOSINE ARABINOSIDE)

Doses of 100-200 mg can be given SQ.

Doses less than 1 gm: Administer via volutrol over 10-20 minutes.

Doses over 1 gm: Administer over 2 hours.

SPECIAL CONSIDERATIONS

Thrombophlebitis, pain at the injection site, should be treated with warm compresses.

Dizziness has occurred with too rapid IV infusions.

Use with caution if hepatic dysfunction exists.

May decrease bioavailability of digoxin when given in combination.

nmc HOMECARE
a division of National Medical Care, Inc.

Diagnosis:

Therapy: Chemotherapy (Cytosine Arabinoside)

Nursing Diagnosis	Goals	Interventions

1. Altered nutrition: less than body requirements related to
A. Nausea and vomiting
   • *Occurs in 50% of patients*
   • *Dose related*
   • *Lasts for several hours*
	1. Pt will be without nausea or vomiting
	2. Nausea and vomiting, if they occur, will be minimal
		1. Premedicate with antiemetics and continue prophylactically 24 hours to prevent nausea and vomiting, at least for first treatment
		2. Assess for s/s of fluid and electrolyte imbalance

B. Anorexia • *Commonly occurs*	3. Pt will maintain baseline wt +/- 5%	3. Encourage small, frequent feedings of favorite foods, especially high-calorie, high-protein (cool, bland foods and liquids if pt. has N/V) 4. Encourage use of spices as tolerated 5. Weekly weights
C. Stomatitis • *Occurs 7-10 days after therapy is initiated in about 15% of pts*	4. Oral mucous membranes will remain intact and without signs of infection	6. Assess oral cavity every day: teach pt to do own oral assessment and oral hygiene regimen and encourage pt to report early stomatitis
D. Diarrhea • *Infrequent and mild*	5. Pt will have minimal diarrhea	7. Encourage pt to report onset of diarrhea, and administer or teach pt to administer antidiarrheal medication

E. Hepatotoxicity • *Usually mild and reversible, but drug should be used cautiously in patients with hepatic dysfunction*	6. Early hepatotoxicity will be identified	8. Monitor LFTs prior to drug dose, especially with high drug doses, assess pt prior to, and during, treatment, for s/s hepatotoxicity
2. Infection and bleeding related to bone marrow depression • *Related to dose and duration of therapy* • *Leukopenic nadir 7-14 days after drug administration; recovery in 3 weeks* • *Thrombocytopenia common* • *Megaloblastic changes in the marrow are common* • *Anemia seen frequently* • *Potent but transient suppression of primary and secondary antibody responses*	1. Pt will be without infection or bleeding 2. S/s of infection or bleeding, if they occur, will be identified early	1. Monitor CBC, platelet count prior to drug administration 2. Assess pt q day for s/s of infection and bleeding 3. Instruct pt in self assessment
3. Alterations in body image, related to Alopecia • *Occurs infrequently*	1. Pt will verbalize feelings re: hair loss, and identify strategies to cope with change in body image	1. Assess pt for s/s of hair loss 2. Discuss with pt impact of hair loss, and strategies to minimize distress; i.e., wig, scarf, cap • *Begin before therapy is initiated*

(continued)

Diagnosis:

Therapy: Chemotherapy (Cytosine Arabinoside)

(continued)

Nursing Diagnosis	Goals	Interventions
4. Potential for injury related to A. Neurotoxicity • *Can occur with high doses* • *Cerebellar toxicity is indication for immediate cessation of therapy* • *Lethargy, somnolence have resulted from too-rapid infusions of drug*	1. Early cerebellar toxicity will be recognized and reported 2. Neurotoxicity will be minimized	1. Assess pt q shift and before administering drug for cerebellar toxicity 2. Instruct pt in self-assessment of cerebellar function. Encourage pt to report changes 3. Report changes in cerebellar function 4. Administer drug according to established guidelines. Monitor pt during infusion for lethargy, somnolence
B. Tumor lysis syndrome (TLS) hyperuricemia • *TLS may develop secondary to rapid lysis of tumor cells* • *Usually begins 1-5 days after initiation of chemotherapy*	3. Serum uric acid, potassium, and phosphorus will remain within normal limits	5. Monitor BUN, creatinine, potassium, phosphorous, uric acid, and calcium 6. Monitor I/O 7. Monitor for renal, cardiac, neuromuscular s/s of TLS 8. Administer allopurinol, fluids as ordered

DRUG

Cisplatin (*Cis*-Platinum, CDDP, Platinum, Platinol)

Class: Heavy metal that acts like alkylating agent

MECHANISM OF ACTION

Inhibits DNA synthesis by forming inter- and intrastrand crosslinks and by denaturing the double helix, preventing cell replication. Is cell cycle phase nonspecific. Has chemical properties similar to that of bifunctional alkylating agents.

METABOLISM

Rapidly distributed to tissues (predominantly the liver and kidneys) with less than 10% in the plasma 1 hour after infusion. Clearance from plasma proceeds slowly after the first 2 hours due to platinum's covalent bonding with serum proteins. 20-74% of administered drug is excreted in the urine within 24 hours.

DOSAGE/RANGE

50-120mg/m^2 every 3-4 weeks
    or
15-20mg/m^2 x5-repeated every 3-4 weeks.

DRUG PREPARATION

10-mg and 50-mg vials. Add sterile water to develop concentration of 1 mg/ml.

Further dilute solution with 250 ml or more of NS or D$_5$W ½ NS. Never mix with D$_5$W, as a precipitate will form.

Refrigerate lyophilized drug, but NOT reconstituted drug, as a precipitate will form.

DRUG ADMINISTRATION

Avoid aluminum needles when administering, as a precipitate will form.

SPECIAL CONSIDERATIONS

Hydrate vigorously before and after administering drug. Urine output should be at least 100-150 ml/hr. Mannitol or furosemide diuresis may be needed to assure this output.

Hypersensitivity reactions have occured, manifested by wheezing, flushing, hypotension, tachycardia. Usually occurs within minutes of starting infusion. Treat with epinephrine, corticosteroids, antihistamines.

Decreases the pharmacologic effects of phenytoin.

Drug causes potasssium and magnesium wasting.

Some ideas to help increase magnesium follow:

To help increase absorption it is recommended that excessive milk, cheese, or other high-calcium products are limited when eating foods high in magnesium.

Calcium and magnesium compete to gain entrance to the body in the intestines, so a high-calcium diet increases requirements for dietary magnesium.

Food high in magnesium: 100 mg or greater per 100 grams.

Nuts:
Almonds
Cashews
Peanuts
Peanut butter
Pecans
Brazil nuts
Walnuts

Other Good Sources:
Whole wheat breads and cereals
Cornmeal
Shredded wheat
Oatmeal
Wheat germ
Brewer's yeast
Cocoa (dry breakfast)
Chocolate (bitter)
Instant coffee and tea
Blackstrap molasses

Peas and Beans:
Split peas
Red beans
White beans

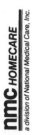

Diagnosis:

Therapy: Chemotherapy (cisplatin)

Nursing Diagnosis	Goals	Interventions

1. Potential alteration in urinary elimination
     • _Drug accumulates in kidney causing necrosis of proximal and distal renal tubules_
     • _Is a dose-limiting toxicity and is cumulative with repeated doses_
     • _Damage to distal renal tubules prevents reabsorption of Mg, Ca, K with resultant decreased serum levels_
     • _Peak detrimental effect usually occurs 10–20 days after treatment and is reversible_
     • _Hyperuricemia may occur due to impaired tubular transport of uric acid but is responsive to allopurinol_
     • _Concurrent use of aminoglycosides is not recommended_
	1. Pt will maintain normal renal functions as evidenced by BUN <20mg/dl, creatinine <1.5mg/dl
	 2. Mg, K,Ca levels will be normal
		1. Prevent nephrotoxicity with vigorous hydration and diuresis to produce urinary output of at least 100 cc/hr
		     • _A typical hydration schedule is NS or 5%D 1/2 NS at 250 cc/hr for 3 hrs prior to cisplatin and for 5 hrs after. Outpatient hydration would be over 1–2 hours. Diuresis is induced by the use of furosemide or mannitol given prior to cisplatin administration_
		 2. Monitor BUN and creatinine prior to initiating drug dose
		     • _Check parameters of BUN and creatinine established in protocol_
		     • _Dose modifications may be made for renal impairment_

2. Altered nutrition: less than body requirements related to
   A. Nausea and vomiting
     • _Nausea and vomiting may be severe; begins 1+ hrs after dose, lasting 8–24 hrs and may recur 48–72 hrs after dose_
	1. Pt will be without nausea and vomiting
	 2. Nausea and vomiting, if they occur, will be minimal
		1. Premedicate with antiemetics and continue prophylactically x 24 hrs to prevent nausea and vomiting, at least for first treatment. Continue antiemetics for 3–5 days
		 2. Encourage small frequent feedings of cool, bland foods and liquids
		 3. Infuse cisplatin over at least 1 hr to minimize

B. Taste Alteration • *Taste alterations can occur with long-term use*	3. Pt will eat adequate calories, proteins, minerals	4. Suggest increased use of spices as tolerated 5. Help pt or significant other develop menu based on past favorite foods 6. Dietary consultation as needed
3. Potential for injury related to anaphylaxis • *Anaphylactic hypersensitivity reactions that have occurred (infrequently) following IV drug administration to previously treated patients: tachycardia, wheezing, hypotension, facial edema* • *Usually controlled by corticosteroids, epinephrine, antihistamines*	1. If anaphylaxis occurs, pt will stabilize	1. Have anaphylaxis tray with corticosteroids, antihistamines, epinephrine ready where chemotherapy is administered • *Discuss with physician the development of standing orders in case anaphylaxis occurs* 2. Monitor and observe patient closely during cisplatin infusions
4. Infection and bleeding related to bone marrow depression • *Bone marrow suppression mild with low to moderate doses* • *High-dose nadir 2-3 weeks with recovery in 4-5 weeks* • *Concurrent low-dose cisplatin with radiotherapy may result in bone marrow suppression*	1. Patients will be without s/s of infection or bleeding	1. Assess pt for s/s of infection and bleeding 2. Monitor CBC, platelet count prior to drug administration
5. Potential for activity intolerance, related to anemia-induced fatigue	1. Pt will be able to do desired activities 2. Early fatigue related to anemia will resolve	1. Monitor hemoglobin, hematocrit. 2. Transfuse per MD for Hct < 25, s/s of severe anemia 3. Teach pt diet high in iron

(continued)

PATIENT CARE PLAN

Diagnosis:

Therapy: Chemotherapy (cisplatin)

(continued)

Nursing Diagnosis	Goals	Interventions
6. Potential for sensory/perceptual alterations related to neurological toxicity • *Neurotoxicity and ototoxicity may be severe* • *Neurotoxicity: glove and stocking distribution with numbness, tingling, and sensory loss in arms and legs* • *Ototoxicity: high-frequency hearing loss above frequency of normal speech, affecting>30% of patients* • *May be preceded by tinnitus* • *Appears dose related and can be unilateral or bilateral* • *Results from the destruction of hair cells that line the organ of Corti* • *Damage is cumulative and may be permanent*	1. Neuropathies and ototoxicities will be identified early 2. If neuropathy occurs, pt will verbalize feelings of discomfort and loss of function and identify alternate coping strategies	1. Assess motor and sensory function prior to therapy • *Baseline audiogram if high-dose cisplatin to be administered* • *Repeat audiogram if pt complains of tinnitus, feeling underwater or auditory discomfort* • *If audiogram reveals hearing decline, discuss with pt and MD benefits/risks of further cisplatin therapy* 2. Encourage pt to verbalize feelings regarding discomfort and sensory loss 3. Help pt discuss alternative coping strategies
7. Potential for sexual dysfunction • *Drug is mutagenic and probably teratogenic*	1. Pt and significant other will understand needs for contraception 2. Pt and significant other will identify strategies to cope with sexual dysfunction	1. As appropriate, explore with pt and significant other issues of reproductive and sexuality patterns, and impact chemotherapy may have 2. Discuss strategies to preserve sexual and reproductive health (i.e., sperm banking, contraception)

Biotherapy Glossary

BIOTHERAPY GLOSSARY

Adoptive Immunotherapy– Cells with antitumor reactivity are administered to a tumor-bearing host and mediate either directly or indirectly the regression of the tumor (e.g., lymphokine activated killer cells or LAK).

Antimetastatic Agents– Agents used to prevent metastases from occurring or to inhibit the ability of cancer cells to grow once the initial metastatic event has occurred (e.g., Laminin).

Biological Response Modifiers– (BRMs, Biologicals)– Agents or approaches that modify the host's biological response to tumor cells with resulting therapeutic benefit.

Colony Stimulating Factor (CSF)– A monokine that stimulates production of leukocytes by stem cells in the bone marrow.

Differentiating Agents– Compounds capable of allowing cancerous or precancerous cells to differentiate or mature to normal cells. (e.g., growth factors, hormones, retinoids.)

Hybridoma– Fusion of a distinct B-lymphocyte clone and an immortal malignant B-lymphocyte yielding large numbers of antibody-secreting cells that are a one clone monoclonal antibody.

Immunomodulator– Agents or approaches that modify components and/or their functions of the immune system in an effort to control or destroy cancerous cells.

Interferon (IFN) – A family of glycoproteins made by mammalian cells in response to viral infections and other types of inducers. They have a variety of biological actions, including antiviral, antiproliferative, antitumor and immunomodulating effects. Alpha, gamma, and beta are three types of interferon.

Interferon Inducer – Agents capable of inducing the release of various types of interferon from the body (e.g., poly ICLC and Sendai virus).

Interleukin-2 (IL-2)– A lymphokine essential to the growth of T-lymphocytes; it augments various T-cell functions and supports the growth and augmentation of natural killer cells.

Lymphokine– a protein secreted by lymphocytes that is capable of directing the function of other cells (e.g., interleukin II, gamma interferon, B-cell growth factor).

Lymphokine Activated Killer Cells– Lymphoid cells capable of lysing either autologous or allogeneic tumor cells.

Monoclonal Antibody– An antibody produced by one single clone of a B-lymphocyte directed against an antigen on tumor cells.

Monokine– A protein secreted by mononuclear phagocytes capable of directing the function of other cells (e.g. alpha interferon, colony stimulating factor, tumor necrosis factor).

Tumor Necrosis Factor (TNF)– A monokine capable of directly killing tumor cells by inducing hemorrhagic necrosis in tumor cells without harming normal tissues.

HANDLING OF CHEMOTHERAPEUTIC AGENTS

Margaret Barton Burke, RN, MS, OCN

HANDLING OF CHEMOTHERAPEUTIC AGENTS
Margaret Barton Burke, RN, MS, OCN

The handling of antineoplastic agents is a concern for practioners working with cancer patients who are receiving chemotherapeutic agents. Practitioners handling antineoplastic agents are exposed to potential health hazards in a variety of settings. Chemotherapy is given in many settings. The home is one of these settings. Potential exposure to antineoplastic agents on a regular basis exists through the preparation and handling of the excreta of patients receiving the drugs. Issues regarding safe handling of these agents have surfaced within the past several years.

The recommendations enclosed in this appendix are based on information from three sources. The first is Cancer Chemotherapy: A Nursing Process Approach by Barton Burke, Wilkes, Berg, Bean, and Ingwersen. (1991 Jones & Bartlett Publishers of Boston, Massachusetts.) The chapter on safe handling contains an extensive review of the literature on safe handling. The second source is Occupational Safety and Health Administration (OSHA). This office publishes recommendations for the handling of cytotoxic agents. These recommendations are approved by the National Study Commission on Cytotoxic Exposure. Finally, the Cetus Corporation has published a wall chart which identifies both in text and graphically the proper handling of cytotoxic agents.

Highlights from all three sources are identified in this appendix. These recommendations are related to care of the cancer patient receiving chemotherapy in the home.

RISKS OF EXPOSURE TO CYTOTOXIC AND HAZARDOUS DRUGS

Primary Routes of Exposure

- Trauma (needle sticks, etc.)
- Inhalation of drug aerosols or droplets
- Absorption through direct skin contact

Procedures that Pose Risk of Exposure During Drug Preparation

- Withdrawal of needles from vials
- Drug transfers using syringes or needles
- Opening ampules
- Expulsion of air from drug-filled syringe
- Changing IV bottles or IV tubing
- Priming IV tubing
- Breakage of vials, IV bottles, etc

Procedures that Pose Risk of Exposure During Drug Administration

- Clearing air from a syringe or IV tubing
  (e.g., priming IV tubing)
- Accidental puncture of a closed system
- Leakage from tubing, syringe, or connection site
- Clipping needles

Procedures that Pose Risk of Exposure During Disposal
of Contaminated Material

- Handling body fluids (blood, excreta, vomitus, ascitic fluid, pleural fluid) of patients who are receiving cytotoxic and hazardous drugs
- Disposal of linens or other materials soaked with body fluids
- Handling spills of cytotoxic and hazardous drugs

PREPARATION AND ADMINISTRATION TECHNIQUES

Before Handling Syringes, IV Bottles, Bags, Ampules, or Vials

- Double gloving is recommended when beginning; surgical latex gloves
- Change outer glove immediately whenever contamination occurs
- Thoroughly wash and dry hands before gloves are donned and when a task is completed

Handling Syringes, Needles, and IV Bottles/Bags

- Use proper aseptic technique
- Properly label all syringes, IV bags, and bottles according to guidelines of policy/procedure manual
- Syringes should be large enough so that they are not full when containing the total drug dose
- Attach and prime drug administration sets within a Biological Safety Cabinet. If available, before drug is added to fluid
- Dispose of used syringes and needles in a puncture-proof container designed for hazardous chemical waste disposal without crushing, clipping or capping

Handling Vials

- Avoid venting medication vials unless using a hydrophobic filter device
- Use Luer-lock type syringe and needle fittings
- Add diluent slowly to the vial by alternately injecting small amounts, allowing air to be displaced
- Maintain negative pressure while withdrawing drug from vial

Handling Ampules

- Tap down any material remaining in the neck and top of an ampule before opening
- Wrap sterile gauze pad around ampule neck before breaking the top
- Keep ampule away from face while opening top
- If diluent is to be added, inject diluent slowly down the inside wall of ampule
- Tilt ampule gently to ensure that all powder is wet before agitating to dissolve contents

Work Practices

- Wash hands before putting on gloves
- Change gowns or gloves immediately if they become contaminated
- Watch infusion sets and pumps for signs of leakage during use; place a plastic-backed absorbent pad under tubing during use to catch any leakage
- Prime the administration set in a Biological Safety Cabinet using a sterile gauze pad; if performed at bedside, use a gauze pad in a plastic bag as a receptacle
- Do not crush or clip used needles and syringes; place in a hazardous chemical waste container
- After administration of drug, place all gauze and alcohol wipes into a hazardous chemical waste container; wash hands upon removal of gloves

SAFETY ISSUES AND WASTE DISPOSAL

Policies and Procedures

- Establish and maintain written policies and procedures for handling cytotoxic and hazardous drugs
- Address personnel issues of conception, pregnancy, and breast feeding in all these policies and procedures
- Include a list of cytotoxic and hazardous drugs in the policies and procedures
- Make policies and procedures easily and readily available to all personnel expected to handle cytotoxic and hazardous drugs
- Make information available on toxicity, treatment of acute exposure, chemical inactivators, solubility, and stability of cytotoxic and hazardous drugs used in the institution/facility

Training and Supervision

- Orientation and training should include:
    - discussion of known and potential hazards of cytotoxic and hazardous drugs
    - explanation of all relevant policies
    - techniques and procedures
    - proper use of protective equipment and materials

- Contents of orientation program and attendance should be well documented and meet "worker right to know" statutes and regulations

Verification and Documentation of Compliance

- Knowledge and competence of personnel preparing and administering cytotoxic and hazardous drugs should be evaluated after initial training and at regular intervals

- Evaulation should include written examination and observed demonstration of competence in preparation and simulated administration of practice solutions

- All personnel involved with cytotoxic and hazardous drugs should be continually updated on new or revised information on safe handling of these drugs

Supplies and Handling

- All heath-care workers who handle cytotoxic and hazardous drugs or waste must be oriented to and must follow procedures governing the identification, containment, collection, segregation, and disposal of cytotoxic and hazardous drug waste materials
- Handle hazardous chemical waste containers with uncontaminated gloves
- Store hazardous chemical waste in labeled, leakproof drums or cartons (in accordance with state and local regulations and disposal contractor's requirements) at a designated area until disposal

Disposal

- All hazardous chemical waste must be segregated from all other trash
- Hazardous chemical waste from drug preparation and patient-care areas should be disposed of as hazardous or toxic waste in an EPA permitted, state licensed hazardous-waste incinerator
- Comply with applicable federal, state, and local regulations regarding disposal

EQUIANALGESIC CHART

Narcotic Oral Equivalent Chart

NARCOTIC ORAL EQUIVALENTS

The importance of pain management for patients with cancer is recognized by oncology nurses, and "alteration in comfort" is a frequent nursing diagnosis with this patient population.

The Narcotic Oral Equivalent Chart was developed to visually display whether a shift from morphine to a morphine equivalent has resulted in an increase or decrease in potency.

Determining the "true" potency of a drug can be especially difficult when patients receive medication that combines a narcotic with a nonsteroidal anti-inflammatory drug such as aspirin or acetaminophen.

The chart ranks medications from the lowest potency of morphine equivalence to the highest. When choosing between different medications, this tool can assist nurses in identifying dosages and making decisions that will prove more beneficial to patients.

Oral Narcotic	IM Morphine Equivalent
Tylenol® #1 (7.5 mg codeine + 300 mg acetaminophen)	1.1 mg
Dilaudid® (hydromorphone 1 mg)	1.3 mg
Codeine 30 mg	1.5 mg
Tylenol® #2 (15 mg codeine + 300 mg acetaminophen)	1.5 mg
Darvon® (propoxyphene hydrochloride 65 mg)	1.6 mg
Darvocet-N® 50 (proyxphene napsylate 50 mg + acetaminophen 325 mg)	1.6 mg
Demerol® (meperidine 50 mg)	1.6 mg
Tylenol #3 (30 mg codeine + 300 mg acetaminophen)	2.3 mg
Percocet® (oxycodone 5 mg + acetaminophen 325 mg)	2.4 mg
Percodan® (oxycodone 5 mg + aspirin 325 mg)	2. 4 mg
Vicodin® (hydrocodone bitartrate 5 mg + acetaminophen 500 mg)	2.9 mg
Tylox® (oxycodone 5 mg + acetaminophen 500 mg)	2.8 mg
Darvocet-N 100 (propoxyphene napsylate 100 mg + acetaminophen 600 mg)	3.1 mg
Morphine 10 mg	3.3 mg
Tylenol #4 (60 mg codeine + 300 mg acetaminophen)	3.8 mg

MORPHINE EQUIANALGESIC LIST

Narcotic Agonists:	IM	P.O	Morphine Equivalent IM
Morphine	1 mg		1.0 mg
	10 mg	30 mg	10.0 mg
	15 mg		15.0 mg
Dilaudid	0.5 mg		4.0 mg
(hydromorphone)	1.0 mg		7.0 mg
	1.5 mg		10.0 mg
	2.0 mg		14.0 mg
		1.0 mg	1.3 mg
		2.0 mg	2.6 mg
		4.0 mg	5.3 mg
		7.5 mg	10.0 mg
Numorphan (oxymorphone)	1.0 mg		10.0 mg
Levo-Dromoran (levorphanol)	2.0 mg	4.0 mg	10.0 mg
Fentanyl (sublimaze)	0.1 mg (100 mcg)		10.0 mg
Dolophine (methadone)	10 mg	20 mg	10.0 mg
Demerol (meperidine)	20 mg		3.0 mg
	25 mg		4.0 mg
	50 mg		7.0 mg
	75 mg	300 mg	10.0 mg
	100 mg		14.0 mg
	125 mg		17.0 mg
Narcotic Mixed Agonist/Antagonists;			
Stadol (butorphanol tartrate)	2 mg		10.0 mg
Buprenex (buprenorphine)	0.3 mg		7.5 mg
	0.4 mg		10.0 mg
Nubain (malbuprine)	10 mg		10.0 mg
	20 mg		15.0 mg
	30 mg		30.0 mg
Talwin (pentazocine)	60 mg		10.0 mg
NSAID:			
Toradol (ketorolac)	30- 90 mg		6-12.0 mg
repeated doses	30 mg		12.0 mg

Based on: Inturrisi, C.E. (1984). Pharmacology of narcotic analgesics. Symposium Management of Cancer Pain. New York: H.P.Publishing Co., Inc., p. 23.

Inturrisi, C.E. (1989). Management of cancer pain- Pharmacology and principles of management. Cancer, 63 (11), 2310-2311.

McCaffery, M. & Beebe, A. (1989). Pain- Clinical Manual for Nursing Practice. St Louis: C.V. Mosby Company, p. 78-79.

PAIN MANAGEMENT PROTOCOL
IN THE HOME

PAIN MANAGEMENT PROTOCOL IN THE HOME

I. According to pain assessment, the following analgesics will be used:

Pain	Analgesic Route	Route	Initial dose/ Frequency
A. Mild (1-2)	Acetaminophen or aspirin or ibuprofen	PO	650 mg q4h ATC 400 mg q4h ATC
B. Moderate/ discomforting (3-4)	Acetaminophen/ codeine (Tylenol #3) Acetaminophen/ hydro- codone (Vicodin or equivalent)	PO PO PO	2 tabs q4h ATC 2 tabs q6h ATC
C. Severe/ distressing (5-7)	Acetaminophen/aspirin /oxycodone (Percodan, Percocet, Tylox)	PO	2 tabs q4h ATC
D. Very severe/ (8-10)	Roxanol concentrate (20 mg/cc) Morphine Sulfate Immediate Release (MSIR) or Hydromorphone (Dilaudid)	PO PO	10-30 mg ATC 4 mg q4h ATC

After 48 h of successful analgesia with MSIR or hydromorphone, or if the patient is already taking strong opioids, may convert to sustained-release morphine (MS Contin or Oromorph).

ATC = Around the clock

II. Constipation Management

	Drug	Dose/frequency	Purpose
A.	Docusate sodium + senna (Senokot-S)	1-2 tabs TID Range: 1 daily to 4 tabs TID	Stool softener
B.	If no bowel movement in 48 hours: Dulcolax	2-3 tabs qHS to TID	stimulant

Rule: one Senokot-S for every 15 mg morphine or its equivalent

III. Nausea Control

Drug	Dose/frequency	Purpose
Prochlorperazine (Compazine)	10 mg PO, R, q4-6h 10 mg spansule q12h 25 mg R suppos q12h 10 mg IM q6h prn	antiemetic
or		
Triethylperazine (Torecan)	10 mg PO, R daily to TID 2 ml IM 1-3 times daily	antiemetic
If gastric stasis, Metoclopramide (Reglan)	10 mg PO q6h (Range: 10 mg q8h to 20 mg q6h)	promote gastric motility

IV. Additional Medications

Drug	Dose/frequency	Purpose
Choline Magnesium Trisalicylate (Trilisate)	1500 mg PO q8-12h	non-narcotic
Ibuprofen (Advil, Motrin)	600 mg PO q6h	prostaglandin inhibitor
Naproxen (Naprosyn)	250-500 mg PO BID	NSAID
Carbamazapine (Tegretol)	200 mg PO BID-QID	neuropathic pain (shooting)
Desipramine (Norpramine)	25 mg HS (10 mg for elderly) Increase by 1 tab q2-3 days until 100-300 mg at HS	neuropathic (burning)
Dexamathasone (Decadron) or Prednisone	Variable	Antiinflammatory
Lorazepam (Ativan) or TID	1 mg PO HS, or titrate from 0.5 to 2 mg BID	anti-anxiety

V. Route

A. ORAL if possible!

B. If dysphagia is present:
   1. Sublingual/ buccal morphine, although not FDA approved, is found to be effective when rectal route is contraindicated; use 1:1 ratio.
   2. Rectal forms of aspirin/acetaminophen/morphine and most anti-emetics are available. Although not approved, sustained-release, oral morphine may be given rectally. Use 1:1 ratio.
   3. Morphine may be administered by subcutaneous infusion. Caregivers must be instructed about management of the pump. Oral to subcutaneous ratio = 3:1.
   4. Intrathecal, epidural, or central line infusions will be considered only if all other routes fail to achieve adequate control.

VI. Guidelines for "rescue doses"

   1. If on sustained-release morphine q12h, supplement with 1/3 of the dose q4h prn.
   2. If 3 or more "rescue doses" are required per 24 hours for break-through pain, total the dose of analgesic per 24 hours and divide into the new around the clock dosing schedule.

Adapted from Northern Illinois Hospice Association, Rockford, IL

TOOLS FOR PAIN ASSESSMENT
OF THE ADULT

PAIN ASSESSMENT CHART
(For Admission and/or Follow-up)

1. Patient _____ 2. DX ____ _____

Assessment on Admission

Date ____ _____   Pain   No Pain   Date of Pain Onset_____

1. Location of Pain (indicate on drawing)

2. Description of Predominant Pain (in patient's words) _____
_____

3. Intensity [Scale 0 (no pain) – 10 (most intense)] _____
_____

4. Duration & when occurs_____
_____
_____
_____

5. Precipitating Factors_____
_____
_____
_____

6. Alleviating Factors_____
_____
_____
_____

7. Accompanying Symptoms

GI: Nausea   Emesis   Constipation   Anorexia

CNS: Drowsiness   Confusion   Hallucinations

Psychosocial: Mood _____ Anger _____
Anxiety_____ Depression _____
Relationships _____

8. Other Symptoms
Sleep_____   Fatigue_____
Activity _____   Other _____

9. Present Medications _____
_____
_____

Doses and times medicated last 48 hours _____
_____

10. Breakthrough Pain _____
_____

Signature:_____

Continuing Pain Assessment and Interventions

Date/ Time																
Med(s)/ Dose																

Most Intense Pain	10																
	9																
	8																
	7																
	6																
	5																
	4																
	3																
	2																
	1																
No Pain Sensation	0																

Blood Pressure																
Respiration																
Nausea																
Emesis																
Constipation																
Anorexia																
Drowsiness																
Confusion																
Hallucinations																
Sleep																
Activity																
Mood																

INSTRUCTIONS: Ask patient to rate the intensity of his/her pain.

Plot this rating on the graph and connect the dots.

Prepared in consultation with Carol P. Curtiss, RN, MSN , and Betty R. Farrell, Ph.D., RN, FAAN, and Alfred McKee, MD.

Visual Analog Scale

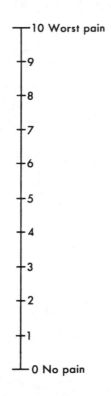

FIGURE 2-4 Vertical visual analog scale. May be duplicated for use in clinical practice. From McCaffery, M. and Beebe, A.: PAIN:CLINICAL MANUAL FOR NURSING PRACTICE, St Louis, 1989. The CV Mosby Company.

Reprinted with permission.

TOOL FOR PAIN ASSESSMENT
OF THE CHILD

PARENT INTERVIEW REGARDING CHILD'S PAIN/HURT

Child:_____

Parent/Caregiver: _____

Date:_____

I. Total Current Situation:

• What are your major concerns (unrelated to pain), if any, about the current situation/hospitalization in general, e.g., finances, care of other children, cause or seriousness of illnesses?

• What are your child's major concerns (unrelated to pain), if any, about the current situation/hospitalization in general, e.g., being separated from parent, sleeping in a different bed or room, missing a birthday party, schoolwork?

II. Child's Previous Experience with Pain/Hurt

• What types of pain has your child had before? Include descriptions of cause, duration, severity, frequency, and other important aspects.

• What words, if any, does your child use for pain or hurt?

• How does your child usually act when he is suddenly hurt, e.g., falls down?

• How does your child usually act when he has been hurting for a long time, e.g., with a sore throat or earache?

III. Assessment of the Child's Current Pain

• Since no one but the child knows if he/she hurts, the health team needs your help in finding out when your child is hurting and whether efforts to relieve the pain are working. What behaviors indicate that your child is or is not in pain right now? For example, can you get your child to smile at you?

• A written record, called a "flow sheet",can be very helpful. What do you suggest be recorded on the flow sheet? List behaviors that probably indicate pain.

• List behaviors that probably indicate comfort.

IV. Comforting the Child and/or Relieving the Pain

• When your child hurts, what do you do to comfort your child or relieve the pain? Which works best? Which could you do now?

• When your child hurts, what does the child do for himself/herself that seems to help? How can we help the child help himself/herself?

• Considering the pain your child has now or will have, what are your concerns about being with your child while he/she is hurting or is undergoing a painful procedure?

• What would you like to learn about how you can soothe or distract your child during pain?

• If painful procedures are performed, do you wish to be with your child? If this wish varies, during which procedures do you wish to be present, and which procedures would you rather avoid?

• Do you have any ideas about how far in advance you child would like to be informed about a painful procedure?

V. Other Comments

• Is there anything special we should know about your child and pain? Is there anything the child finds disturbing that we should not do?

• Reprinted with permission from McCaffery, M; Beebe, A. *Pain: a clinical manual for nursing practice.* St. Louis, MO: The C.V. Mosby Company, 1989:272-273.

WONG/BAKER FACES RATING SCALE

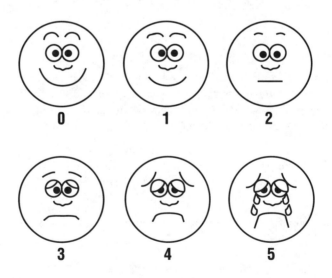

1) Explain to the child that each face is for a person who feels happy because he has no pain (hurt, or whatever word the child uses) or feels sad because he has some or a lot of pain.

2) Point to the appropriate face and state, "This face is...":

0—"very happy because he doesn't hurt at all."
1—"hurts just a little bit."
2—"hurts a little more."
3—"hurts even more."
4—"hurts a whole lot."
5—"hurts as much as you can imagine, although you don't have to be crying to feel this bad."

3) Ask the child to choose the face that best describes how he feels. Be specific about which pain (e.g."shot" or incision) and what time (e.g. now? earlier before lunch?).

From Wong, D., and Whaley, L.: Clinical Handbook of Pediatric Nursing, ed 2, p. 373, St. Louis, 1986, The C.V. Mosby Company. Printed with permission of the publisher and authors who also give their permission for this to be duplicated and used in the care of children with pain.

Wong/Baker Faces Rating Scale (can be duplicated for use in clinical practice).

COMPLICATION MANAGEMENT/TROUBLESHOOTING OF VASCULAR ACCESS DEVICES

COMPLICATION MANAGEMENT/TROUBLESHOOTING
of VASCULAR ACCESS DEVICES

Complication/Problem Experienced	Troubleshooting	Possible Causes
Unable to withdraw blood Able to infuse 'one-way valve' (most common problem reported)	• Change patient position, have patient deep breath, cough, standup, walk around.	• Migration of catheter into smaller vessel catheter tip against vessel wall.
	• Check position of Huber needle.	• Huber needle not fully advanced thru septum.
	• Flush gently with 10-20 ml NS to assure catheter function.	• Fractured catheter between clavicle and first rib.
		• Damaged catheter in subcutaneous tunnel.
	• If unsure consider chest x-ray/ venogram catheter may need to be repositioned under fluoroscopy.	
	• Flush in push/pull manner with 10-20 ml NS to dislodge Fibrin sleeve or intralumen clot.	• Temporary/ Fibrin sleeve or intralumen clot.
	• Use Fibrinolytic agent (urokinase 5000 u) in a volume slightly.	

Signs/Symptoms	Interventions	Possible Causes
Unable to infuse or withdraw.	greater than that of catheter. Follow instructions carefully. • Chest x-ray/venogram. • Consider continuous infusion of fibrinolytic agent. • Removal of catheter/device. • Check position of Huber needle. • Use Fibrinolytic agent (as above). • Use push/pull motion.	• Thrombophlebitis with clot formation along catheter. • Extensive thrombosis. • Huber needle not fully advanced thru septum. • Intralumen clot. • Drug precipitation (Heparin & non-compatible drug). • Catheter kinked or in knot.
Arm edema, swelling of neck. Enlarged superficial vein of chest.	• Chest x-ray/venogram. • Removal of catheter/device.	• Extensive thrombosis. • Superior vena cava syndrome.
Infection Local	• Re-evaluate site care.	• Poor technique used for site care. • Patient may be sensitive to betadine. • Needle in too long/not secured well.

COMPLICATION MANAGEMENT/TROUBLESHOOTING OF VASCULAR ACCESS DEVICES

Complication/Problem Experienced	Troubleshooting	Possible Causes
	• If drainage present–take culture. • Daily meticulous site care. • No occlusive dressings until infection resolves. • Use topical antibiotics as indicated. • Removal of port needle. • Do not use port until symptoms resolve. • If sutures involved– remove. Secure catheter end–resuture when symptoms resolve. • If symptoms do not resolve device may have to be removed.	
Systemic Fever, chills, diaphoresis, gastric symptoms Headache, malaise Hyperventilation Hypotension Muscle aches Weakness Oliguria Mental status	• D/C infusion/change • Blood culture — from catheter — from peripheral vein • Course of IV antibiotics through device. • Over wire exchange of catheter if possible. • If infection continues to reoccur device may need to be removed.	• Contaminated infusate • Contaminated hub, insertion site, etc. • Non-Catheter related sepsis.

Reference: Herbst, S. *Care of the HIV Patient with a Vascular Access Device, In: Lewis, Angie (Ed.) Nursing Care of the Patient with AIDS/ARC, Aspen, 1988.*

DEGREES OF HYPERCALCEMIA:
SIGNS AND SYMPTOMS

DEGREES OF HYPERCALCEMIA: SIGNS AND SYMPTOMS *

Body System Affected	Mild (less than 12 mg/dL)	Moderate (12-15 mg/dL)	Severe (Above 15 mg/dL)
Gastrointestinal	anorexia, nausea, vomiting, vague abdominal pain	constipation, increased abdominal pain, abdominal distension	atonic ileus, obstipation
Neurologic	restlessness, difficulty in concentrating, depression, apathy, lethargy, clouding of consciousness	confusion, psychoses, somno-lence	coma———>death
Muscular	easily fatigued, muscle weakness (generalized or involving shoulders and hips), hyporeflexia	increased muscular weakness, bone pain	profound muscular weakness, ataxia, pathologic fractures
Renal	nocturia, polyuria, polydipsia	renal tubular acidosis, renal calculi	oliguric renal failure, renal insufficiency, azotemia
Cardiovascular	hypertension (may or may not be present)	cardiac dysrhythmias, EKG abnormalities (shortening of QT interval on EKG, coving of ST-T wave, widening of T wave)	cardiac arrest———>death

*Signs and symptoms regardless of serum calcium levels may vary from person to person
Reprinted with permission by the publisher from Poe, C.M. & Radford, A. I. (1985). The challenge of hypercalcemia in cancer. Oncology Nursing Forum, 12 (6): 31.

1983 METROPOLITAN HEIGHT AND WEIGHT TABLES

1983 METROPOLITAN HEIGHT AND WEIGHT TABLES

According to Height and Frame, Ages 25 and Over
Weight (in indoor clothing)

WOMEN

Height in shoes Feet	Inches	Cm.	Small Frame Lb.	Kg.	Medium Frame Lb.	Kg.	Large Frame Lb.	Kg.
4	10	147	102-111	46-50	109-121	49-55	118-131	54-60
4	11	150	103-113	47-51	111-123	50-56	120-134	55-61
5	0	152	104-115	47-52	113-126	51-57	122-137	55-62
5	1	155	106-118	48-54	115-129	52-59	125-140	57-64
5	2	158	108-121	49-55	118-132	54-60	128-143	58-65
5	3	160	111-124	50-56	121-135	55-61	131-147	59-67
5	4	163	114-127	52-58	124-138	56-63	134-151	61-69
5	5	165	117-130	53-59	127-141	58-64	137-155	62-70
5	6	168	120-133	55-60	130-144	59-65	140-159	64-72
5	7	170	123-136	56-62	133-147	60-67	143-163	65-74
5	8	173	126-139	57-63	136-150	62-68	146-167	66-76
5	9	175	129-142	59-64	139-153	63-69	149-170	68-77
5	10	178	132-145	60-66	142-156	64-71	152-173	69-79
5	11	180	135-148	61-67	145-159	66-72	155-176	72-80
6	0	183	138-151	63-69	148-162	67-74	158-179	72-81

1983 METROPOLITAN HEIGHT AND WEIGHT TABLES

According to Height and Frame, Ages 25 and Over
Weight (in indoor clothing)

MEN

Height in shoes Feet	Inches	Cm.	Small Frame Lb.	Kg.	Medium Frame Lb.	Kg.	Large Frame Lb.	Kg.
5	2	158	128-134	58-61	131-141	59-64	138-150	63-68
5	3	160	130-136	59-62	133-143	60-65	140-153	64-70
5	4	163	132-138	60-63	135-145	61-66	142-156	64-71
5	5	165	134-140	61-64	137-148	62-67	144-160	65-73
5	6	168	136-142	62-64	139-151	63-69	146-164	66-74
5	7	170	138-145	63-66	142-154	64-70	149-168	68-76
5	8	173	140-148	64-67	145-157	66-71	152-172	69-78
5	9	176	142-151	64-69	148-160	67-73	155-176	70-80
5	10	178	144-154	65-70	151-163	69-74	158-180	72-82
5	11	180	146-157	66-71	154-166	70-75	161-184	73-84
6	0	183	149-160	68-73	157-170	71-77	164-188	74-85
6	1	185	152-164	69-74	160-174	73-79	168-192	76-87
6	2	188	155-168	70-76	164-178	74-81	172-197	78-90
6	3	191	158-172	72-78	167-182	76-83	176-202	80-92
6	4	193	162-176	74-80	171-187	78-85	181-207	82-94

ASSESSMENT GUIDE TO
ORAL AND PHYSICAL CONDITIONS

AN ASSESSMENT GUIDE TO
ORAL AND PHYSICAL CONDITIONS

Numerical and Descriptive Ratings

Variable	1	2	3	4
Lips	smooth, soft, moist to dry	rough, dry, may be crusted	rough, swollen, dry, may be blistered	dry, cracked, bleeding, or ulcerated
Mucous membranes, palates, oropharynx	pink, moist, no debris	red, edematous, slightly dry, burning sensation	red, dry, may be ulcerated or coated with debris	very red or ulcerated, inflamed, probable debris
Gingivae	pink, moist, no debris	pale, slightly dry, may have reddened areas or pustules	red, shiny, edematous, ulcerated	red, shiny, ulcerated, bleeds easily
Teeth	shiny, no debris	slightly dull, some debris	dull, debris clinging to 1/2 of the visible enamel	very dull, covered with debris
Dentures	well-fitting	slightly loose	loose with areas of irritation	cannot be worn due to irritation

Tongue	pink, moist, no fissures or prominent papillae	dry, pink with red areas or coated with no red areas, medial groove deepened, papillae prominent	dry, swollen, entire tongue red but tip, coated at base, papillae all over tongue are raised, giving a peppered appearance	very dry with indentations, tip is very red, sides are blistered, coating extends to tip or tongue is deeply grooved and thickened
Saliva	thin and watery	increased in amount	scanty, mouth dry	thick and ropy, viscid
Ability to swallow	swallows/eats with no problem	discomfort on swallowing/eating	pain on swallowing/eating	unable to swallow/eat
Diet	normal in fluid and amount of chewing needed	little chewing needed, soft, blenderized, or liquid	NPO with tube feedings or total parenteral nutrition	NPO with intravenous fluids only
Breathing	via nose and mouth without help, normal rate	mouth breathing, increased rate	uses oxygen or airway	tracheostomy, ventilator, or endotracheal tube
Self-care	independent	needs to be encouraged to eat and do oral hygiene	assistance needed to eat and do oral hygiene	totally dependent on others for eating and oral hygiene

Adapted from: S. Beck. "Impact of a Systematic Oral Care protocol on Stomatitis after Chemotherapy." Cancer Nursing 2 (June 1979): p. 192. Copyright held by Masson Publishing USA, INC.

Reprinted with permission by the editor from Ziga, S.E. (1983). Stomatitis/Mucositis, in J.M. Yasko (ed) Guidelines for Cancer Care: Symptom Management. Published by Reston Publishing Co, Inc. Copyright held by Joyce M Yasko.

ANTIEMETICS COMMONLY USED
WITH CHEMOTHERAPY

ANTIEMETICS COMMONLY USED WITH CHEMOTHERAPY - RELATED NAUSEA AND VOMITING

	AVAILABILITY	RECOMMENDED DOSE/SCHEDULE	SIDE EFFECTS/COMMENTS
Phenothiazines Prochlorperazine (Compazine®)	Soln: 5mg/ml; tabs: 5, 10, 25 mg; sustained release (Compazine® spansules): 10, 15, 30 mg; suppositories: 2.5, 5, 25 mg; parenteral 5 mg/ml	"Low" dose: 10 mg p.o./IM, 25 mg PR q 4 hrs. or 1/2 hrs AC & HS "High" dose: 20-40 mg slow IV 30 min. before, 3 hrs. and 6 hrs. after chemo For delayed N&V; 30 mg TID day 1*, 30 mg BID day 2*, 15 mg BID days 3 thru 6 *plus dexamethanasone	Most common s.e.: EPS (akathisia and dystonic rxn) and sedation - children more prone to EPS -dehydration may increase risk of akathisia -treat akathisia with benzodiazepine (diazepam or lorazepam) -treat dystonic rxn with diphenhydramine or benztropine Hypotension may occur, particularly with 1st parenteral dose -do not exceed 5 mg/min. with IV dose -administer IV doses of >10 mg over 20-30 min. to recumbent patient -hypotension and other CV effects (i.e., tachycardia) usually resolve within 1/2-2 hrs -monitor VS Other common side effects: CNS (drowsiness, anxiety, HA, etc) Anticholinergic (dry mouth, constipation, etc.) -Use SR capsules on regular basis for delayed/persistent N&V

Thiethylperazine (Torecan®)	Tabs: 10 mg; suppositories: 10 mg; parenteral: 5 mg/ml	10 mg q 4 hr.	See prochlorperazine for side effects
Perphenazine (Trilafon®)	Tabs: 2, 4, 8, 16 mg; parenteral: 5 mg/ml	4 mg po q 4-6 hrs. 5-10 mg IM q 4-6 hrs. For intractable vomiting; dilute to 0.5 mg/ml and give IV at rate of not more than 1 mg over 1-2 min, not to exceed 5 mg.	Similar to prochlorperazine Off label use for intractable vomiting: 5 mg IV bolus followed by cont IV infusion of 1 mg/hr until vomiting controlled
Butyrophenones Haloperidol (Haldol®)	Soln: 2 mg/ml; tabs: 0.5, 1, 2, 5 mg; parenteral: 5 mg/ml	Doses Variable: 1 mg BID-TID PRN; 2mg IM; 3 mg IV q 2 hrs x 5 Starting 30 min. prior to chemotherapy	Use lowest effective dose. Similar in structure to phenothiazines; may be as effective May have additive effects with other CNS depressants, i.e., opioid analgesics, sedatives, barbituates Side effects: EPS (treat as with phenothiazines), sedation, tachycardia, hypotension, anticholinergic
Droperidol (Inapsine®)	Parenteral 2.5 mg/ml (IM, IV)	Doses Variable: 1mg IVP q hr. x 6; 15 mg IV, then 7.5 mg IV q 2 hrs x 7	See haloperidol Sedation may persist for up to 12 hrs Hypotension: consider hypovolemia -monitor I&O -monitor VS -administer IV fluids PRN

(continued)

ANTIEMETICS COMMONLY USED WITH CHEMOTHERAPY - RELATED NAUSEA AND VOMITING

	AVAILABILITY	RECOMMENDED DOSE/SCHEDULE	SIDE EFFECTS/COMMENTS
Substituted Benzamide Metoclopramide (Reglan®)	Soln: 5 mg/ml; tabs: 5 mg, 10 mg; parenteral: 5 or 10 mg/ml	2-3 mg/kg IV or p.o. q 2-3 hr x 3-5; 3 mg IV 30 min before and 90 min after chemo; 2 mg/kg/ p.o. or IV q 2hrs x 3, then 1 mg/kg q 2hrs x 3	Administer IV doses slowly (over 15 min.) to prevent transient, intense anxiety Compatible with dexamethasone in IV soln May have additive effects with other CNS depressants Side Effects: EPS -treat as with phenothiazines -more common in children, adolescents and young adults -more common with p.o. administration over several days Sedation, HA, fatigue, restlessness, diarrhea, decreased renal plasma flow -monitor I&O -monitor VS
Steroids Dexamethasone (Decadron®) Methylprenisolone (Solu-Medrol®)		Doses Variable: methylpred-nisolone 500 mg IV q 6hrs x 4 dexamethasone 10-20 mg IV prior to chemo; dexamethasone 80-150 mg IV x 1; dexamethasone 20 mg IV x 6 2 hrs before chemo and 3, 6, 9, and 12 hours post chemo	Rapid IV administration may be accompanied by transient perineal, rectal, or vaginal burning Side Effects: insomnia, anxiety, euphoria

	dexamethasone 8 mg p.o. TID day 1, 8 mg BID day 2, and 4 mg BID days 3-6 for delayed N&V	
Cannabinoid Dronabinol (Marinol®)	Tabs: 2.5, 5, 10 mg 5 mg/kg q 4-6 hrs.	Schedule II drug, generally used as second line antiemetic Side Effects; CNS-sedation, dizziness, disorientation, impaired concentration, anxiety, dysphoria ANS-orthostatic hypotension, dry mouth CV-tachycardia

(continued)

ANTIEMETICS COMMONLY USED WITH CHEMOTHERAPY - RELATED NAUSEA AND VOMITING

	AVAILABILITY	RECOMMENDED DOSE/SCHEDULE	SIDE EFFECTS/COMMENTS
Benzodiazepine Lorazepam (Ativan®)	Tabs: 0.5, 1, 2 mg (p.o. or sublingual); parenteral: 2 or 4 mg/ml	Doses variable: 0.5-2 mg p.o. or IV x 1 or repeat PRN; 1.5 mg/m^2 IV before chemo (3 mg max); 0.025 mg/kg before chemo (4 mg max) and q 4hrs PRN x 4; 0.025 mg/kg sublingual before chemo	Sublingual provides rapid plasma levels and greater bioavailability than p.o. administration Side effects: sedation, amnesia May have additive effect with other CNS depressants, i.e., opioids, sedatives, etc. Use cautiously in patients with hepatic or renal dysfunction (organs of metabolism & excretion) Use cautiously in debilitated patients or those with compromised pulmonary function (may lead to underventilation and hypoxia) -monitor labs -monitor VS -monitor LOC -administer small dose and repeat to desired effect
5-HT Blocker Ondansetron (Zofran®)	parenteral: 2 mg/ml multidose vial	0.15 mg/kg q 4 hrs x 3 doses. Give first dose 1/2 hr before chemo	Dilute in 50 ml 5% dextrose soln or 0.9% saline soln & give IV over 15 min. Delayed N/V 24 hrs after chemo; need to have patient take alternate antiemetic during that time, as drug is only approved for three - dose use.

Adapted with permission from Wickham, R. (1989). Managing chemotherapy-related nausea and vomiting: The state of the art. Oncology Nursing Forum, 16 (4): 566-8. Copyright held by Oncology Nursing Press, Inc.

GONADAL DEVELOPMENT & PSYCHOLOGICAL THEMES POST-BONE MARROW TRANSPLANT

TABLE 8

Gonadal Development Post-transplant

Growth Phase	BMT Treatment	Gonadal Development
Prepubertal	Chemotherapy	Develop normal through puberty • possible child-bearing • low/normal sperm count • temporary impotence
	Chemotherapy/TBI	Delayed secondary sex characteristics • body hair • genitalia size • growth spurt • breast development • menstruation • high pitched voice in males • temporary impotence
Postpubertal	Chemotherapy	Return to normal gonadotrophin levels • temporary impotence

	Chemotherapy/TBI	Gonadal failure
		Female
		    • estrogen production ceased
		    • early menopause
		    • atrophy of genitalia
		    • vaginal dryness
		    • sterility
		Male
		    • temporary impotence
		    • sterility

TABLE 9

Psychological Themes Experienced in Discharge Phase of Post-BMT

Patient

Fear of leaving protected environment
Re-entry into family/society
Changes in body image
Fear of being emotional/financial burden
Insurance/employment discrimination
Fear of recurrent disease
Changes in relationships
Loss of or change in sexual identity
Profound fatique
Relief from completion of treatment
Survival guilt
Change in life priorities/perspectives
Age regression/dependency
Situational stress

Specific to Children

Sibling rivalry
Restricted activity levels
Difficulty with re-entry into school

Family

Fear of leaving protected environment
Fear of caring for patient at home
Caregiver burnout
Finances
Fear of recurrent disease
Changes in relationships
Alteration in intimacy
Relief from completion of treatment
Change in life priorities/perspectives
Situational stress